HISTORY OF CERVICAL CANCER AND THE ROLE OF THE HUMAN PAPILLOMAVIRUS, 1960–2000

The transcript of a Witness Seminar held by the Wellcome Trust Centre for the History of Medicine at UCL, London, on 13 May 2008

Edited by L A Reynolds and E M Tansey

Volume 38 2009

First published by the Wellcome Trust Centre
for the History of Medicine at UCL, 2009

The Wellcome Trust Centre for the History of Medicine
at UCL is funded by the Wellcome Trust, which is
a registered charity, no. 210183.

ISBN 978 085484 123 3

All volumes are freely available online following the links to Publications/Wellcome Witnesses at
www.ucl.ac.uk/histmed

CONTENTS

ILLUSTRATIONS AND CREDITS

ABBREVIATIONS*

ABC	'**A**chievable standards, **B**enchmarks for reporting, **C**riteria for evaluating cervical cytopathology' (Herbert (ed.) (1995); Johnson (ed.) (2000))
AIDS	acquired immune deficiency syndrome or acquired immunodeficiency syndrome
ARTISTIC	A Randomized Trial In Screening To Improve Cytology (Sargent *et al.* (2008))
BECC	British Empire Cancer Campaign (Cancer Research Campaign from 1970)
BMS	biomedical scientists
BPV	bovine papillomavirus
BSCC	British Society for Clinical Cytology (1961)
BSCCP	British Society for Colposcopy and Cervical Pathology (1972)
CIN	cervical intraepithelial neoplasia
CIS	carcinoma *in situ*
CRPV	cotton-tail rabbit papillomavirus
CSP	NHS Cervical Screening Programme
DNA	deoxyribonucleic acid
GVS	Gynaecological Visiting Society of Great Britain and Ireland (1911)
HART	HPV in addition to routine testing study (Cuzick *et al.* (2003))
HPV	human papillomavirus
HSV	herpes simplex virus
IARC	International Agency for Research on Cancer
IBMS	Institute of Biomedical Science (formerly the Institute of Medical Laboratory Technology/Science)

* Details in parentheses refer to previous name, date of foundation or reference to classic paper

ICRF	Imperial Cancer Research Fund
LBC	liquid-based cytology
MRC	Medical Research Council
NHS CSP	NHS Cervical Screening Programme
NICE	National Institute for Health and Clinical Excellence (formerly National Institute for Clinical Excellence)
p53	*protein 53* or *tumour protein 53*
PCR	polymerase chain reaction
RCGP	Royal College of General Practitioners
RCOG	Royal College of Obstetricians and Gynaecologists
RCPath	Royal College of Pathologists
RLU	relative light units
RNA	ribonucleic acid
SCMR	standardized cohort mortality ratios
SMR	standardized mortality ratio
STI	sexually transmitted infection
TOMBOLA	Trial of Management of Borderline and Other Low-Grade Abnormal smears (Cotton *et al.* (2006))
VLPs	virus-like particles

WITNESS SEMINARS: MEETINGS AND PUBLICATIONS[1]

In 1990 the Wellcome Trust created a History of Twentieth Century Medicine Group, associated with the Academic Unit of the Wellcome Institute for the History of Medicine, to bring together clinicians, scientists, historians and others interested in contemporary medical history. Among a number of other initiatives the format of Witness Seminars, used by the Institute of Contemporary British History to address issues of recent political history, was adopted, to promote interaction between these different groups, to emphasize the potential benefits of working jointly, and to encourage the creation and deposit of archival sources for present and future use. In June 1999 the Governors of the Wellcome Trust decided that it would be appropriate for the Academic Unit to enjoy a more formal academic affiliation and turned the Unit into the Wellcome Trust Centre for the History of Medicine at UCL from 1 October 2000. The Wellcome Trust continues to fund the Witness Seminar programme via its support for the Centre.

The Witness Seminar is a particularly specialized form of oral history, where several people associated with a particular set of circumstances or events are invited to come together to discuss, debate, and agree or disagree about their memories. To date, the History of Twentieth Century Medicine Group has held more than 50 such meetings at the time of publication, most of which have been published, as listed on pages xiii–xvii.

Subjects are usually proposed by, or through, members of the Programme Committee of the Group, which includes professional historians of medicine, practising scientists and clinicians, and once an appropriate topic has been agreed, suitable participants are identified and invited. This inevitably leads to further contacts, and more suggestions of people to invite. As the organization of the meeting progresses, a flexible outline plan for the meeting is devised, usually with assistance from the meeting's chairman, and some participants are invited to 'set the ball rolling' on particular themes, by speaking for a short period to initiate and stimulate further discussion.

---

[1] The following is the standard introductory text to the *Wellcome Witnesses to Twentieth Century Medicine* series.

Each meeting is fully recorded, the tapes are transcribed and the unedited transcript is sent to every participant. Each is asked to check his or her own contributions and to provide brief biographical details. The editors turn the transcript into readable text, and participants' minor corrections and comments are incorporated into that text, while biographical and bibliographical details are added as footnotes, as are more substantial comments and additional material provided by participants. The final scripts are then sent to every contributor, accompanied by forms assigning copyright to the Wellcome Trust. Copies of all additional correspondence received during the editorial process are deposited with the records of each meeting in archives and manuscripts, Wellcome Library, London.

As with all our meetings, we hope that even if the precise details of some of the technical sections are not clear to the non-specialist, the sense and significance of the events will be understandable. Our aim is for the volumes that emerge from these meetings to inform those with a general interest in the history of modern medicine and medical science; to provide historians with new insights, fresh material for study, and further themes for research; and to emphasize to the participants that events of the recent past, of their own working lives, are of proper and necessary concern to historians.

ACKNOWLEDGEMENTS

'History of Cervical Cancer and the Role of the Human Papillomavirus, 1960–2000' was suggested as a suitable topic for a witness seminar by Professor David Jenkins, who assisted us in planning the meeting. We are very grateful to him for that input and to Professor Glenn McCluggage for his excellent chairing of the occasion. We are particularly grateful to Professor Anne Johnson for writing the Introduction to the published proceedings. Our additional thanks go to Professor Leopold Koss, Dr Arthur Spriggs and Dr Nasseem Husain, who have allowed us to reproduce some of their reminiscences in Appendices 1 and 2. We thank the participants for their help with the Glossary and Dr Lionel Crawford, Professor Leopold G Koss and Mrs Marilyn Symonds for help with photographs. For permission to reproduce other images included here, we thank the Banbury Center of Cold Spring Harbor Laboratory Archives, the British Society for Clinical Cytology and Ms Beth Moore. Professor Valerie Beral did not assign copyright for the use of her contribution and thus it is included as reported speech.

As with all our meetings, we depend a great deal on staff of the Wellcome Trust to ensure their smooth running: especially the audiovisual, catering, reception and security departments and Wellcome Images. Mr Akio Morishima supervised the design and production of this volume; Ms Liza Furnival provided the index; and Mrs Sarah Beanland and Mr Simon Reynolds read the transcript for sense and consistency; and Ms Stefania Crowther has given editorial and marketing assistance. Mrs Jaqui Carter transcribed the tapes, and Mrs Wendy Kutner and Ms Stefania Crowther assisted in running the meeting. Finally we thank the Wellcome Trust for supporting this programme.

Tilli Tansey

Lois Reynolds

Wellcome Trust Centre for the History of Medicine at UCL

VOLUMES IN THIS SERIES*

1. **Technology transfer in Britain: The case of monoclonal antibodies**
   Self and non-self: A history of autoimmunity
   Endogenous opiates
   The Committee on Safety of Drugs (1997)
   ISBN 1 86983 579 4

2. **Making the human body transparent: The impact of NMR and MRI**
   Research in general practice
   Drugs in psychiatric practice
   The MRC Common Cold Unit (1998)
   ISBN 1 86983 539 5

3. **Early heart transplant surgery in the UK (1999)***
   ISBN 1 84129 007 6

4. **Haemophilia: Recent history of clinical management (1999)**
   ISBN 1 84129 008 4

5. **Looking at the unborn: Historical aspects of obstetric ultrasound (2000)**
   ISBN 1 84129 011 4

6. **Post penicillin antibiotics: From acceptance to resistance? (2000)**
   ISBN 1 84129 012 2

7. **Clinical research in Britain, 1950–1980 (2000)***
   ISBN 1 84129 016 5

8. **Intestinal absorption (2000)***
   ISBN 1 84129 017 3

9. **Neonatal intensive care (2001)**
   ISBN 0 85484 076 1

*Volumes in print and freely available from Dr Carole Reeves, see page xvi.

10. **British contributions to medical research and education in Africa after the Second World War (2001)**
ISBN 0 85484 077 X

11. **Childhood asthma and beyond (2001)***
ISBN 0 85484 078 8

12. **Maternal care (2001)**
ISBN 0 85484 079 6

13. **Population-based research in south Wales: The MRC Pneumoconiosis Research Unit and the MRC Epidemiology Unit (2002)**
ISBN 0 85484 081 8

14. **Peptic ulcer: Rise and fall (2002)***
ISBN 0 85484 084 2

15. **Leukaemia (2003)***
ISBN 0 85484 087 7

16. **The MRC Applied Psychology Unit (2003)***
ISBN 0 85484 088 5

17. **Genetic testing (2003)***
ISBN 0 85484 094 X

18. **Foot and mouth disease: The 1967 outbreak and its aftermath (2003)***
ISBN 0 85484 096 6

19. **Environmental toxicology: The legacy of *Silent Spring* (2004)***
ISBN 0 85484 091 5

20. **Cystic fibrosis (2004)**
ISBN 0 85484 086 9

21. **Innovation in pain management (2004)**
ISBN 978 0 85484 097 7

22. **The Rhesus factor and disease prevention (2004)**
ISBN 978 0 85484 099 1

23. **The recent history of platelets in thrombosis and other disorders (2005)**
ISBN 978 0 85484 103 5

24. **Short-course chemotherapy for tuberculosis (2005)**
ISBN 978 0 85484 104 2

25. **Prenatal corticosteroids for reducing morbidity and mortality after preterm birth (2005)**
ISBN 978 0 85484 102 8

26. **Public health in the 1980s and 1990s: Decline and rise? (2006)**
ISBN 978 0 85484 106 6

27. **Cholesterol, atherosclerosis and coronary disease in the UK, 1950–2000 (2006)**
ISBN 978 0 85484 107 3

28. **Development of physics applied to medicine in the UK, 1945–1990 (2006)**
ISBN 978 0 85484 108 0

29. **Early development of total hip replacement (2007)**
ISBN 978 0 85484 111 0

30. **The discovery, use and impact of platinum salts as chemotherapy agents for cancer (2007)**
ISBN 978 0 85484 112 7

31. **Medical ethics education in Britain, 1963–1993 (2007)**
ISBN 978 0 85484 113 4

32. **Superbugs and superdrugs: The history of MRSA (2008)**
ISBN 978 0 85484 114 1

33. **Clinical pharmacology in the UK, *c.* 1950–2000: Influences and institutions (2008)**
ISBN 978 0 85484 117 2

34. **Clinical pharmacology in the UK, *c.* 1950–2000: Industry and regulation (2008)**
ISBN 978 0 85484 118 9

35. **The resurgence of breastfeeding, 1975–2000 (2009)**
ISBN 978 0 85484 119 6

36. **The development of sports medicine in twentieth-century Britain (2009)**
ISBN 978 0 85484 121 9

37. **History of dialysis, *c.* 1950–1980 (2009)**
ISBN 987 0 85484 122 6

38. **History of cervical cancer and the role of the human papillomavirus, 1960–2000 (2009)**
ISBN 987 0 85484 123 3 (this volume)

39. **Clinical genetics in Britain: Origins and development (2010)**
ISBN 987 0 85484 127 1 (in press)

40. **The medicalization of cannabis (2010)**
ISBN 987 0 85484 129 5 (in press)

All volumes are freely available online at www.ucl.ac.uk/histmed following the links to Publications/Wellcome Witnesses.

*Volumes freely available, while stocks last, from Dr Carole Reeves at: c.reeves@ucl.ac.uk

Hard copies of volumes 21–38 can be ordered from www.amazon.co.uk; www.amazon.com; and all good booksellers for £6/$10 each plus postage, using the ISBN.

UNPUBLISHED WITNESS SEMINARS

1994 **The early history of renal transplantation**

1994 **Pneumoconiosis of coal workers**
(partially published in volume 13, *Population-based research in south Wales*)

1995 **Oral contraceptives**

2003 **Beyond the asylum: Anti-psychiatry and care in the community**

2003 **Thrombolysis**
(partially published in volume 27, *Cholesterol, atherosclerosis and coronary disease in the UK, 1950–2000*)

2007 **DNA fingerprinting**

The transcripts and records of all Witness Seminars are held in archives and manuscripts, Wellcome Library, London, at GC/253.

OTHER PUBLICATIONS

Technology transfer in Britain: The case of monoclonal antibodies
Tansey E M, Catterall P P. (1993) *Contemporary Record* **9**: 409–44.

Monoclonal antibodies: A witness seminar on contemporary medical history
Tansey E M, Catterall P P. (1994) *Medical History* **38**: 322–7.

Chronic pulmonary disease in South Wales coalmines: An eye-witness account of the MRC surveys (1937–42)
P D'Arcy Hart, edited and annotated by E M Tansey. (1998) *Social History of Medicine* **11**: 459–68.

Ashes to Ashes – The history of smoking and health
Lock S P, Reynolds L A, Tansey E M. (eds) (1998) Amsterdam: Rodopi BV, 228pp. ISBN 90420 0396 0 (Hfl 125) (hardback). Reprinted 2003.

Witnessing medical history. An interview with Dr Rosemary Biggs
Professor Christine Lee and Dr Charles Rizza (interviewers). (1998) *Haemophilia* **4**: 769–77.

Witnessing the Witnesses: Pitfalls and potentials of the Witness Seminar in twentieth century medicine
Tansey E M, in Doel R, Søderqvist T. (eds) (2006) *Writing Recent Science: The historiography of contemporary science, technology and medicine.* London: Routledge: 260–78.

The Witness Seminar technique in modern medical history
Tansey E M, in Cook H J, Bhattacharya S, Hardy A. (eds) (2008) *History of the Social Determinants of Health: Global Histories, Contemporary Debates.* London: Orient Longman: 279–95.

Today's medicine, tomorrow's medical history
Tansey E M, in Natvig J B, Swärd E T, Hem E. (eds) (2009) *Historier om helse* (*Histories about Health,* in Norwegian). Oslo: Journal of the Norwegian Medical Association : 166–73.

INTRODUCTION

It took nearly 150 years from Rigoni-Stern's observation that 'cancer of the uterus' might be related to sexual lifestyle (page 83), for Human Papilloma Virus (HPV) to be established as the cause of cervical cancer in the 1980s. His observation that cancer was more common in married women than virgins and nuns in nineteenth-century Verona gave the first clue to aetiology. A century later epidemiological studies identified the sexual behavioural risks for cervical cancer in both women and their male partners. In parallel, gynaecologists, virologists and cytologists were making rapid advances in their understanding of the natural history of cervical cancer, the detection through cervical cytology of preinvasive stages of cervical cancer, and we're beginning to explore the possibility of a viral cause.

This Witness Seminar volume gives fascinating insights into the science, serendipity, and dogged commitment of a generation of clinicians, virologists, cytologists, epidemiologists, and public health specialists in establishing cervical screening as a sensitive, specific and effective tool to reduce cancer mortality. Papanicolaou developed his smear test for early cancer detection in 1943 but it took until 1988 for a properly organised population-based service to be established in England.

The witnesses here trace the work leading to the discovery of HPV as a cause of cervical cancer through advances in detection methods which identified oncogenic viral types and thus paved the way for development of HPV vaccines.

But with the evolution of the science comes the determined and tireless effort of those who drove screening policy (such as Muir Gray, Jocelyn Chamberlain and Catherine Pike), those gynaecologists who were early adopters (such as Stanley Way and later Albert Singer) and the army of major contributors (mainly women) who led and executed the programmes of screening, read the smears, improved the accuracy and standardization of methods of sample collection, cytological protocols, call and recall and clinical follow-up over the course of several decades.

I have not been directly involved in cervical cancer research but have followed the unfolding story of aetiology and control from the sidelines over the last 30 years with gratitude for what has been achieved. It is my generation who were among the first to benefit from cervical cancer screening and it will be my daughter's generation who will be the first hopefully to benefit from the introduction of HPV vaccination. But like the cervical screening programme before it, population benefit will only be achieved through high uptake and efficacy against all the predominant circulating oncogenic viruses.

I first became aware of the beginnings of cervical screening in the 1960s. Both my parents were gynaecologists and worked for Stanley Way in Newcastle in the 1940s and 1950s. My mother recounts details of the radical surgery undertaken by Way for advanced case of cancer and the early experiments comparing outcomes of surgery and radium treatment, but mortality was high.[2]

Accounts of the 1960s and 1970s abound with tales of the uncertainty about effectiveness of screening and the disorganization, inconsistency and opportunistic nature of much screening. Lamentably much of that uncertainty might have been circumvented if Archie Cochrane's calls for randomized clinical trials had been heeded (pages 18 and 59, notes 44 and 162).

My mother, along with many women doctors of her generation, was in part-time work in family planning and cervical cytology clinics. She lamented the poor technique used by many doctors and recalls teaching the importance of visualization of the cervix to local GPs in Manchester, and the days of undertaking screening of women in factories around Manchester in a mobile unit. But she felt her efforts detected more ovarian than cervical pathology. Too often they were screening the low-risk women.

Her account resonates with the report here. The 1960s and 1970s were the years of concerted effort to improve the specificity and consistency of tests and the coverage of screening by those who were the product champions of the day. While attempts had been made by the then Ministry of Health to establish a smear testing programme in 1964, it was not until 1988 that the current NHS Cervical Screening Programme was established, largely as an outcome of the efforts of the 1987 Intercollegiate Working Party (pages 26–9). An impassioned editorial in the *Lancet*, attributed to George Knox, is testimony to the frustration felt about the lack of substantial impact on cancer mortality between 1964 and 1984 at least in part, because of the lack of an organised population-based approach: 'No-one knows what proportion of women have been screened at different ages, and what proportion have not.'[3]

---

[2] My mother still has an unpublished report of Way's travels to Canada and the US in the early 1950s, where he recounts some of the early cytology being carried out there. These documents, along with other records of the meeting, will be deposited at GC/253 in archives and manuscripts, Wellcome Library, London.

[3] Anon (1985): 363.

There are parallels with another sexually transmitted infection, *Chlamydia trachomatis,* in which an 'opportunistic' screening programme is currently being 'rolled-out', among young men and women, without randomized controlled trial (RCT) evidence of effectiveness, and without population coverage or defined screening interval. In the week in which I write, a report for the National Audit Office raised concerns about lack of uptake or evaluation of outcomes and poor value for money.[4]

Assessing effectiveness of the programme relied on observational data of rates of cervical cancer and cancer deaths. But as Sasieni set out (page 64), it was difficult to assess impact because it was known that cervical cancer incidence and cervical intraepithelial neoplasia (CIN) 3 were increasing in those born after 1940. Beral described this in her *Lancet* article of 1974. In an elegant analysis based on standardized cohort mortality ratios (SCMRs), she was able to demonstrate that SCMRs at age 20 in successive birth cohorts from 1902–47 rose and fell in parallel with changing incidence of gonorrhoea. Risk was highest among women whose husbands were in occupations associated with higher sexually transmitted infection (STI) risk (pages 31–2).[5]

The putative changes in sexual behaviour driving the growing gonorrhoea epidemic from the 1960s to the mid-1980s (when AIDS resulted in a rapid decline in incidence) were not documented in population studies until 1990. The first National Survey of Sexual Attitudes and Lifestyles (Natsal), of which I was principal investigator, was famously banned from public funding by Margaret Thatcher and later funded by the Wellcome Trust.[6] The study documented the rapid decline in age at first intercourse from the 1950s onwards, the rising rate of sexual partner change driving the observed increase in STI incidence and, as we now know, the underlying silent epidemic of oncogenic HPV infection. No wonder, with incidence of the underlying cause rising, that it was difficult to demonstrate any major impact of incomplete screening on cervical cancer mortality. But mortality rates did decline substantially after 1988.[7]

---

[4] National Audit Office (2009). Summaries available at www.nao.org.uk/publications/0809/young_peoples_sexual_health.aspx. For news coverage of the report, see http://news.bbc.co.uk/1/hi/health/8354932.stm (both sites visited 24 November 2009).

[5] Beral (1974).

[6] Johnson *et al.* (1992, 1994). A Witness Seminar on 'The history of the National Sexual Attitudes and Lifestyles Survey' will be held on 14 December 2009 and will be published as volume 41 in the *Wellcome Witnesses to Twentieth Century Medicine* series.

[7] Sasieni and Adams (1999).

The idea that cervical cancer was associated with some aspect of sexual lifestyle was not new in the 1960s and Stanley Way and later Albert Singer and others were among those who studied the 'male factor' in the aetiology of cervical cancer. The idea that it might be related to a specific viral infection was gathering strength (pages 29–32).

In retrospect, the initial suggestion of Herpes Simplex Virus (HSV) as a cause of cervical cancer by Rawls *et al.* in 1968 diverted attention from HPV, a classical case of association being confused with causality.[8] A range of STIs could be associated with cervical cancer because they shared the common route of sexual transmission. But the HSV hypothesis held sway through much of the 1980s, despite the failure to demonstrate viral DNA in malignant tissue (page 34).

This Witness Seminar report has something of the air of a detective story, with strands of evidence from different disciplines all contributing to the identification of the aetiological role of HPV. The recognition that the koilocytes were similar to cells from histological condylomata contributed to the identification of HPV in these cells. The development of virological methods in the 1970s identified the different types of HPV, followed by the discovery by Gissman and zur Hausen of HPV16 and 18 in 1980.[9] Methods of hybrid capture assays and polymerase chain reaction all revolutionized detection, characterization, and quantification of infectious organisms, and knowledge of their role in health and disease. As Patrick Walker attests, it took some time before the 'received wisdom' that HSV had a role in cervical cancer aetiology could be put to rest (pages 33–4). It seems that only in the last decade with the successful development of HPV vaccines, that HPV has been generally accepted as a cause.

The importance of the work of the late Jian Zhou with Ian Frazer in developing the underlying virological work which made the production of a vaccine possible is given due emphasis in the transcript (pages 43–6). It has arguably been a gratifyingly short time between the discovery of HPV as a cause of cervical cancer and the implementation of a vaccination programme in young women. The debate will continue about the scientific and economic factors underpinning the choice in the UK of a bivalent rather than quadrivalent vaccine as in the US and Europe,[10] and thus will likely extend to the value of vaccinations in males.[11]

---

[8] Rawls *et al.* (1968).

[9] Gissmann and zur Hausen (1980).

[10] Kmietowicz (2008).

[11] Castle and Scarinci (2009).

It will need another generation to measure the population uptake of vaccine and impact on cervical cancer, since the vaccine will not protect against all oncogenic viruses. The cervical screening programme will in turn need to be re-evaluated in successive cohorts. It is too early to measure the longer term acceptability and uptake of the current vaccine, which has had its proponents and detractors. Public concerns about vaccine safety will always cause nervousness among policy and programme leaders. The death of a young woman in 2009 shortly after receiving HPV vaccination was subsequently shown to be unrelated to the vaccine, but was sufficient to suspend the UK programme for a few days until the cause of death was known.[12]

The well organized population-based cervical screening programme established since 1988 has demonstrated its impact through secondary prevention of cervical cancer. The impact of the primary prevention programme through HPV vaccination on future generations is the culmination of a fascinating scientific story and one for future historians to recount.

Anne M Johnson
Division of Population Health and Institute for Global Health, UCL

[12] O'Dowd (2009).

HISTORY OF CERVICAL CANCER AND THE ROLE OF THE HUMAN PAPILLOMAVIRUS, 1960–2000

The transcript of a Witness Seminar held by the Wellcome Trust Centre for the History of Medicine at UCL, London, on 13 May 2008

Edited by L A Reynolds and E M Tansey

HISTORY OF CERVICAL CANCER AND THE ROLE OF THE HUMAN PAPILLOMAVIRUS, 1960–2000

Participants

Professor Valerie Beral
Professor Saveria Campo
Professor Jocelyn Chamberlain
Professor Dulcie Coleman
Dr Lionel Crawford
Professor Heather Cubie
Professor Jack Cuzick
Dr Ian Duncan
Dr Winifred Gray
Dr Amanda Herbert
Professor David Jenkins
Dr Elizabeth Mackenzie
Dr Joan Macnab
Professor Glenn McCluggage (chair)
Professor Anthony Miller
Professor Julian Peto
Dr Catherine Pike
Professor Peter Sasieni
Professor Albert Singer
Dr John Smith
Professor Margaret Stanley
Mrs Marilyn Symonds
Dr Anne Szarewski
Dr Tilli Tansey
Professor Leslie Walker
Mr Patrick Walker
Dr Margaret Wolfendale
Professor Ciaran Woodman

Among those attending the meeting: Mr Ken Campbell, Professor Steve Gallivan, Ms Rosemary Sowerby, Dr Elizabeth Toon, Dr David Wright

Apologies include: Dr Malcolm Anderson, Professor Leszek Boryseiwicz, Professor Xavier Bosch, Dr Peter Boyle, Professor Linda Bryder, Dr Blanche Butler, Professor Nicholas Day, Dr John Doorbar, Professor Harold Fox, Dr Sylvia Franchesci, Professor Dr Lutz Gissmann, Sir Muir Gray, Professor Sir Andrew Haines, Dr O A N (Nasseem) Husain, Dr Jane Johnson, Professor Joe Jordan, Professor Henry Kitchener, Professor Ilana Loewy, Professor Attila Lörincz, Mr Michael Palmer, Mrs Julietta Patnick, Professor Frank Sharp, Professor Peter Stern, Professor Sir James Underwood, Professor David Whynes, Mr Dennis Williams

Dr Tilli Tansey: I would like to begin by welcoming you to this Witness Seminar on cervical cancer and the human papillomavirus from 1960 to 2000. These Witness Seminars were started by the Wellcome Trust about 15 years ago and they are designed to get together a group of people who have been involved in a particular event or discovery, or people who have seen a lot of changes in their professional lives, to get them together to talk and discuss among themselves, sometimes disagree quite drastically, about what happened and why did things happen. We all know that if we read conventional scientific papers and medical accounts, it doesn't always tell us how things happened and why. So that is the purpose of these meetings. The entire meeting is recorded and transcribed and then the transcript is edited and published.

Because we are going to record everything, we would like people to contribute informally as the meeting goes on. Nothing will be published without your permission, so we will ask you to assign legal copyright to the Wellcome Trust. This meeting was suggested by Professor David Jenkins, who is now an affiliated worker in the Wellcome Trust Centre for the History of Medicine at UCL, where he is working on this subject. We are delighted that Professor Glenn McCluggage from Belfast, who is a consultant pathologist there, has agreed to be our chairman for this meeting. So without further ado, I will hand over to Glenn.

Professor Glenn McCluggage: Good afternoon everyone, and welcome to this Witness Seminar. Probably most of you in this audience don't know me, but I am a gynaecological histopathologist in Belfast and I suspect everybody in this audience knows more about HPV than myself. My interest in HPV started quite a few years ago. I started off in gynaecological pathology by reporting a lot of cervical punch and loop biopsies[1] from colposcopy clinics and so I see a lot of disease related to human papillomavirus and it is certainly a very important topic to be discussed. Hopefully, my role will be limited. It is either making sure that the discussion keeps going or, on occasions, to stop people talking who are going on for too long.

You have a list of topics that we will try to discuss and the format is going to be fairly open regarding each of these (Table 1).[2] Without further ado, I am going to introduce Professor David Jenkins, who is going to set the scene. David worked in the University of Nottingham for many years and had a very

---

[1] See Glossary, page 145.

[2] A general draft outline of each Witness Seminar is circulated among all participants prior to the meeting. The outline is flexible and not all the topics listed are covered in depth. See Table 1, page 4.

Cervical cytology and colposcopy
How did cervical cytological screening develop
Who became a cytologist and why
Life and interactions in a cervical screening laboratory
The impact of colposcopy in the 1980s
The discovery of HPV and development of HPV research
'The unknown male factor'
Finding HPV 16 and 18
The mechanisms and genes of HPV
p53 and VLPs
Immune responses to HPV
Epidemiology and the natural history and importance of HPV
The UK national screening programme
Evidence on when screening works and when not
The organization of a national programme and the screening centers
The public health impact of screening reorganization
Later developments in applying understanding of HPV
HPV testing
HPV testing in triage and screening
The personal dimension

Table 1. Outline programme for 'The History of Cervical Cancer and the Role of the Human Papillomavirus, 1960–2000' Witness Seminar

firm interest in preinvasive cervical lesions, and latterly he has been working in Brussels, helping to organize clinical trials with one of the new HPV vaccines. So David, could you start us off?

Professor David Jenkins: First of all, may I welcome everybody. It's great that people have come. The gestation of this meeting has been around about two years, so it's taken a while to contact everybody, to get everything established and to actually be able to hold this meeting. Thanks to Tilli Tansey and the Wellcome Trust for sponsoring and organizing the meeting and to Professor McCluggage for chairing it. It's very important that the chairman is not an HPV person, because we need somebody, who is not too deeply involved as a protagonist in HPV, to be a neutral chairman for this session.

My interest in this subject goes back a long way, and one of the attractions of HPV and cervical cancer for me is that it is a microcosm of relationships between science, medicine and society. A lot of key issues that are involved in the interactions between these different worlds are brought out in the study of HPV and cervical cancer, in the development of cervical screening and more recently now with the vaccines for preventing HPV infection and thus cervical cancer.[3] We have decided to cut this discussion off at 2000 because we don't really want to get too much into the current controversies in which many people are still involved, and the areas where there are still big decisions to make.

We want to look at how two parallel stories have developed: one is the evolution of cervical cancer prevention through screening, and the second is the HPV story since the early 1960s, since cervical screening was first introduced then, and how these two have become intertwined in relation to attempts to prevent cervical cancer. This has also had a lot of spin-offs. It has meant that it has been a very multidisciplinary activity, there are a lot of different people involved, and I am glad that we have been able to get a good mixture of cytologists, pathologists, clinicians, epidemiologists, psychologists, as well as a few medical historians involved in this meeting.

It is a really interesting area, and one of the fascinating parts of it is the way in which it has grown up as an area in the era of sex, drugs, and rock and roll. Certainly we all know that sex has been heavily involved in HPV transmission, but it is a different sexually transmitted disease from the conventional ones. Some of the issues that have happened and affected HPV have seen people trying to draw parallels with traditional sexually transmitted diseases and particularly with HIV, as another new disease, but a very different one.

The history that we want to get today, as Tilli has said, is a bit of the unofficial history, as well as people's role in the official history of the development of both screening and HPV. We don't want to indulge in conventional hagiography of some kinds of medical history. When I was researching this, I looked through what was available on the web about George Papanicolaou and there's some stuff which really amounts to almost canonization of the guy. He was born in the same town as an ancient physician, Diocles (who was second only to Hippocrates), and he looked after a leper colony, arrived penniless in the US and, in order to begin to fund his academic activities, worked as a rug salesman, while his wife worked as a tailor. That's wonderful, and may or may not be totally true, but we want to get to some of the more ordinary stories, and some of the actual ways in which this admittedly important initial step with screening was translated into the huge success of cervical screening by thousands of people – doctors,

[3] The UK national programme to vaccinate girls aged 12–13 years began in September 2008, along with some girls aged 17 years, using the bivalent vaccine *Cervarix* (GSK) giving protection against HPV subtypes 16 and 18; girls aged 16–18 years were eligible from September 2009; and those aged 15–17 years of age from September 2010. See Anon (2008); Gilman *et al.* (2009).

public health workers, technicians and screeners in many countries and very successfully in the UK. We also know that the HPV story has expanded from very small numbers of people in the 1970s and 1980s, up to the International Papillomavirus Conferences and International Papillomavirus Society meetings, which regularly attract over 1000 people every 18 months.[4]

McCluggage: Shall we consider how cervical cytology screening developed?

Dr Elizabeth Mackenzie: It is good to see so many of my colleagues from the past here, the great, the good and the not so good. It does give me great pleasure to be here.

I had an interesting beginning: I trained at Bart's in the dim and distant past, qualified in 1957, and when we got back to England from Malta in 1961, I think it was my husband, Campbell, who decided that there was no way that I was ever going to get a job and that I ought to do public health, which is what I duly did. I am eternally grateful, because I think that's the thing that made me understand what screening was all about.[5] It wasn't taking smears and forgetting about them. From there I got up to Glasgow, with five sessions a week. The gynaecologist in Glasgow asked: 'Would I like to do a closed community survey of the women in Campbeltown?', which is where Campbell came from and it certainly is closed.[6] I went to get trained and my first mentor was Helena Hughes.[7] So I trained and set up the beginnings of the screening programme in the Southern General Hospital in Glasgow, but then, like all dutiful wives, moved down to London in 1967. I was introduced to Dr Nasseem Husain,

---

[4] For an evaluation of the early history of cytodiagnosis, and the final page of Papanicolaou's 1928 paper, see Spriggs (1977): 1094. See also Papanicolaou and Traut (1943); Traut and Papanicolaou (1943); Fremont-Smith and Graham (1952). Dr Margaret Wolfendale wrote: 'To make the historical context more comprehensive it might be worth mentioning that as a result of Aureli Babeş independently recognizing that cervical cancer could be recognized in cervical smears in Bucharest in 1927, this test was routinely used on a large scale by Kermauner and Schiller (Spriggs (1977)).' Note on draft transcript, 26 November 2008. See Babeş (1931); see also note 239.

[5] Dr Elizabeth Mackenzie wrote: 'Mr James Mair, one of the more enlightened gynaecologists, suggested that it would be useful to train in cytology with Helena Hughes at the Glasgow Royal Infirmary and set up a screening programme in the small isolated town of Campbeltown in Kintyre. Dr Elizabeth Macgregor had already established a very successful well-organized screening programme covering the population of Aberdeen.' Note on draft transcript, 26 November 2008.

[6] Dr Elizabeth Mackenzie wrote: 'This remained a paper exercise only, as we returned south to England.' E-mail to Mrs Lois Reynolds, 13 September 2009.

[7] See, for example, Evans *et al.* (1986, 1987).

my second mentor, in a very busy laboratory at St Stephen's Hospital, Chelsea, who I thought was going to be here today. It was the first time I learned about automatic screening.[8] He seemed to think that a bit of kit from Cambridge Instruments – a densitometer – was going to automatically screen the smears, which was absolute nonsense, because they were not monolayered cells. It was terrific fun and I had some lovely papers out of that.[9]

I then moved to Bristol in 1969, and the one thing about being a trained cytologist was that you got a job anywhere. The hospitals were desperately short. I then started up in Bristol, which was a moderate sized town of about 400 000, and there the beginnings of my interest in screening programmes started.[10] This business about 'you can't take smears and forget about it,' is not possible.

We had the chief accountant of the South West Electricity Board as chairman of Southmead Hospital board, who was interested in computers.[11] We were then taken over by the area health authority, and, I must say, it was really interesting persuading our colleagues that women didn't need to be screened at five-minute

[8] Dr Husain was unable to attend the Witness Seminar on 13 May 2008. Dr Elizabeth Mackenzie wrote: 'Dr Nasseem (O A N) Husain was experimenting with automated screening using normally prepared smears, but attempting to identify malignant cells by their staining densities. Unfortunately it took some years for this to progress and it wasn't until the introduction of the preparation of monolayered samples that this was successful. It is interesting to note that in contrast to Scotland, England was training non-medical staff to undertake primary screening. Despite having no previous scientific training, many of them provided the major staffing in the screening laboratories and their contribution was later recognized by the British Society for Clinical Cytology (BSCC) with a diploma and, for the more senior, membership of the society.' Note on draft transcript, 26 November 2008. See, for example, Husain (1972).

[9] See, for example, Husain *et al.* (1970); Spriggs (1969). Further details of the Quantimet image analyser with densitometer can be found at www.computerhistory.org/brochures/companies.php?alpha=g-i&company=com-42bc1cec137d6 (visited 30 April 2009).

[10] Dr Elizabeth Mackenzie wrote: 'I worked with Dr Frank Lewis in Bristol and it is interesting to note that none of my mentors started out with an interest in gynaecological cytology; Helena Hughes, Nasseem Husain and Frank Lewis were a gynaecologist and two haematologists, respectively.' Note on draft transcript, 26 November 2008.

[11] Dr Elizabeth Mackenzie wrote: 'Interestingly, the development of the computer programme in Bristol was supported by the chairman of Southmead Hospital board. His son persuaded his firm, IBM, to provide us with computer expertise and suitable software to screen the Avon population of 250 000 women between the ages of 20 and 64 every five years. The five-year interval programme in Bristol proved to be successful and it prevented unnecessary interval smears from overloading the laboratory, as we returned them to the sender unread if there were no clinical signs or symptoms. This policy was unpopular to begin with until it was realized that it was effective and there was a finite amount of money supporting the service.' Note on draft transcript, 26 November 2008.

intervals; you could have a reasonable sort of screening service at five-yearly intervals, although I might add that several people here will disagree with me, and certainly at that stage it was quite a miracle to get a regular screening interval. The other thing was to get it into proper records, so that wherever these women went, their screening histories followed them.[12]

Jenkins: That's a good introduction, because, I think, it raises a lot of important points about the start of screening, mainly how disorganized it was.

Mackenzie: May I say one thing about screening in Scotland? What was interesting about Scotland is that they trained doctors to screen, and the only good thing that I got out of it was that you knew exactly what screening was all about, you didn't treat it lightly. Your colleagues who were screeners and eventually everyone in the screening service deserved enormous support and pats on the back.[13] It was a very different set-up in Scotland, which was all doctor-led, which was a so-called 'waste of expertise'. I think the combination of screeners and medical people in the screening service made a huge difference to what went on.

Jenkins: So when did you start using screeners in the screening service?

Mackenzie: We had screeners from day one when I got to Bristol in 1969. I think it was quite a while before they started using screeners in Scotland.[14]

Dr Ian Duncan: The initial screeners in Scotland in the early 1960s were, as Liz Mackenzie has pointed out, enthusiastic female doctors. There was Elizabeth Macgregor in Aberdeen, Helena Hughes in Glasgow, and Helen Duguid in Dundee.[15] They employed part-time female doctors largely, and this was because, of course, the nature of screening meant that you had to do it part-time. You couldn't spend all day screening, because you can't maintain that

---

[12] For further discussion about the *Lancet* 1985 editorial, see pages 14 and 19. See also Threlfall *et al.* (1997).

[13] See also notes 8, 21, 24 and pages 8–9, 22–23.

[14] Dr Euphemia McGoogan set up the BSCC national certificate of competence in cytology screening examination (end-of-training exam for cytology screeners) in 1988 and ran it for three years. She co-authored the NHS Cervical Screening Programme (NHSCSP) training logbook for cytology screeners and designed a logbook and training programme for trained cytology screeners wishing to gain competence in reading liquid-based cytology cervical samples. See www.csi.org.nz/proceedings/mcgoogan.pdf (visited 30 September 2009).

[15] See Dr Elizabeth (Betty) Macgregor's Biographical note, page 136.

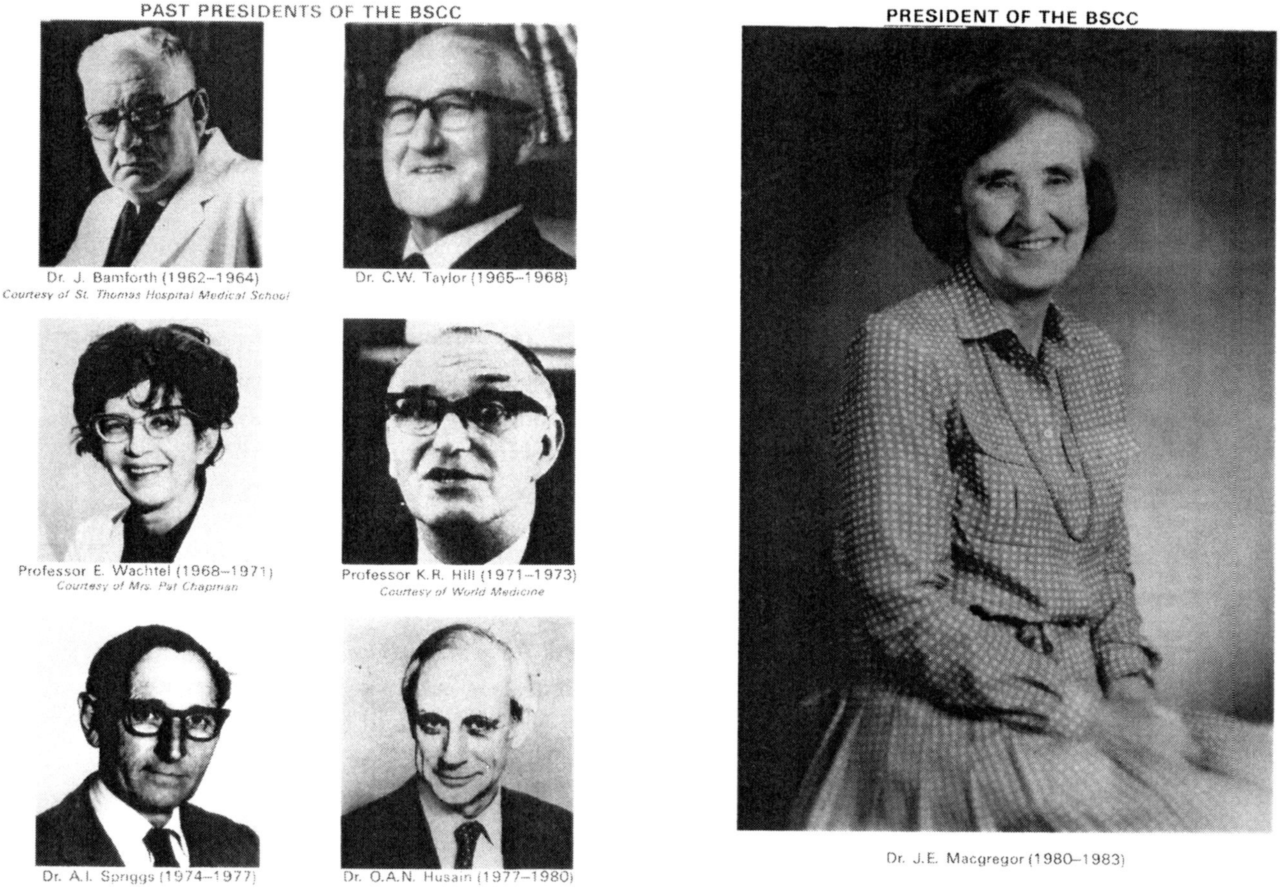
PAST PRESIDENTS OF THE BSCC
Dr. J. Bamforth (1962–1964)
Courtesy of St. Thomas Hospital Medical School
Dr. C.W. Taylor (1965–1968)
Professor E. Wachtel (1968–1971)
Courtesy of Mrs. Pat Chapman
Professor K.R. Hill (1971–1973)
Courtesy of World Medicine
Dr. A.I. Spriggs (1974–1977)
Dr. O.A.N. Husain (1977–1980)
PRESIDENT OF THE BSCC
Dr. J.E. Macgregor (1980–1983)

Figure 1: Presidents of the British Society for Clinical Cytology (BSCC), 1962–83.
BSCC (1983): 2–3.

level of concentration. It very much suited the individual who didn't want to devote the whole day to medical work. I think that the cytoscreeners then were laboratory technicians, and that was the way that they trained, as laboratory technicians. They then became screeners themselves, again, very much on a part-time basis, and that happened in the late 1960s–early 1970s.

Dr Margaret Wolfendale: I started in cytology in 1962 and there are quite a few parallels, because I became a cytologist as I had moved with my husband.[16] In those days there was very, very little open to women in medicine, unless they were going to dedicate their whole life to it, full-time. The only part-time work was either as an assistant in general practice, or else in family planning. I was working at the Royal Marsden Hospital, Fulham, as a junior registrar with Dr Humphrey Kay in the Fetal Tissue Bank and I didn't want to move when my husband moved to the country.[17] At the time there was an article written by Geoffrey Crabbe and Mary Egerton in the *BMJ*, talking about cytology.[18] I went to my old hospital, the Royal Free, to train and then wrote round, it was an awful cheek really, saying I had done some cytopathology and did anybody want a cytopathologist in the Northampton, Aylesbury, Luton or Bedford areas. At the time, it was the Oxford region, which was one of the forefront regions employing married women, that took me on as a cytopathologist and my mentor was Arthur Spriggs.[19] I started a lot of the district general hospital cytopathology in the Oxford region under his supervision.

Jenkins: One of the things that intrigues me about the very early days of cytology is that it really wasn't organized in any national sense, or in any sense above that which was generated by the consultants themselves.[20] It would be nice to

---

16 See also Dr Elizabeth Mackenzie's discussion on page 6.

17 Lawler (1981).

18 Dr Margaret Wolfendale wrote: 'Crabbe and Egerton (1961) was one of a spate of publications on this topic in 1961.' Note on draft transcript, 26 November 2008.

19 See Biographical note on page 140–1; see also Figure 1, page 9.

20 Dr Margaret Wolfendale wrote: 'Arthur Spriggs aptly pointed out that the "emergence of a body of trained exfoliative cytologists" resulted in population screening becoming an accepted practice before the general introduction of randomized controlled trials with the result that it became "a football between public health authorities, epidemiologists, lay pressure groups, politicians and clinical cytologists" (Spriggs (1977): 1095, 1096). Max Wilson, who worked at the DHSS at the time and was a great proponent of cervical screening, was of the opinion that "in the early 1960s mainly on the evidence of pathology… the time when a (randomized controlled) trial…could be considered ethical had by then passed" (Wilson (1971): 71).' Note on draft transcript, 26 November 2008.

hear a bit more about that: how people organized their own local screening programmes.

Professor Dulcie Coleman: I would like to talk a little bit about that and how disorganized it was. In about 1964 the then Ministry of Health agreed that cervical smear tests should be offered, to be available, to every woman.[21] There were really no formal plans of how this should be done, but every pathologist became responsible for this. I think there were four or five training schools set up, and that's important to record, because these were very important.[22] I know there was Erica Wachtel[23] and Chandra Grubb in London, Betty Attwood in Birmingham[24] and Blanche Butler in Manchester. One sort of offered oneself to these schools for training; there seemed to be no special funding for it, but

[21] The Ministry of Health's 1964 circular announced the introduction of a series of training courses in exfoliative cytology open to pathologists and medical laboratory technicians, as a result of the Standing Medical Advisory Committee recommendation that revision of cytological facilities in hospital pathology should be accelerated. The cervical cytology service was established in 1965, offering five-yearly smears to all women over the age of 35 years. The National Archives, Kew, holds files on the early development of screening (MH154/46–48). For further discussion of the efficacy of the training courses, see Wilson (1967); for later reports, see Farmery and Gray (1994); House of Commons, Committee of Public Accounts (1992). See also note 33.

[22] Five training schools to teach cytodiagnosis were set up in 1964 at the Hammersmith Hospital, London, the Royal Free Hospital, London, Birmingham, Manchester and Newcastle. For current arrangements, see www.cancerscreening.nhs.uk/cervical/training.html (visited 29 July 2009). The BSCC included training sessions in their scientific meetings, description of which can be found in BSCC (1983): 25–62.

[23] Dr Erica Wachtel (d. 1980) was at the Postgraduate Medical School, Hammersmith Hospital in 1961. See also Wachtel and Plester (1952, 1954); Figure 1.

[24] Mrs Marilyn Symonds wrote: 'In 1952 a meeting at the Royal College of Obstetricians and Gynaecologists, attended by Birmingham gynaecologist Professor Hugh McLaren, suggested sending two medics to visit Dr Papanicolaou in the US to study his technique for cervical cancer detection. Miss M E Attwood (Betty), a young technician working in the university department in Birmingham, was sent instead, as Professor McLaren and Dr Claude Taylor (pathologist) thought a technical person would be more appropriate to learn the technique. Betty left six weeks later by boat from Southampton and worked for 18 months with Papanicolaou in New York. She then worked at the Free Hospital in Boston followed by time in Florida working with Ayre (of the Ayre spatula). She returned to Birmingham and set up a research cervical screening routine, screening 2500 women. The results of this study were written up (Attwood *et al.* (1956); McLaren *et al.* (1958)), but no-one took much notice. They continued to screen women and eventually obtained funding to set up one of the first UK cytology training schools in Birmingham in the early 1960s. It was part of the medical school and eventually moved to the maternity hospital. Betty continued to run the training school together with Dennis Williams until her retirement. As a result of her early work she was often invited to speak at meetings all over the world and has been involved in writing several research papers.' E-mail to Mrs Lois Reynolds, 11 September 2009; see also Figure 2, page 13.

that was the way to get your training, and that was the way that I got mine, with Erica Wachtel. It was fairly basic training, because you were shown slides, and told: 'This is abnormal and this isn't'.[25] There was no one to explain to you what you were looking at or to explain that the aim of the exercise was to detect a precancerous condition. This was in the early days of training. That was one aspect.

Another aspect was that there was a preponderance of women in cervical cytology. Many of the pathologists, who were responsible for offering or arranging screening in their own hospitals, really were not in a position to cope with the job because it is very time-consuming, and they were willing to take on anyone. I remember saying: 'Well, I have been to a training school', like Margaret had, and 'I know how to do it.' They said: 'All right, we will take you on a trial basis.' You were put in a little hole in the corner to get on with it on your own. I remember I actually sat in a fireplace, my feet were in the fireplace, and my microscope was on the mantelpiece and I had a suitably high stool to sit on.[26] Until I proved my worth, I wasn't given an office or a proper desk or anything. This is the way it started up. But it evolved from there and now there is a very well-organized training programme and training is very carefully monitored, and, I am proud to say, there is even academic training offered, an MSc course which started in 1990, at St Mary's Hospital Medical School (now part of Imperial College London) and continues to be offered today.[27] We have come a long way from those early days.

Professor Albert Singer: You mentioned exclusively female screeners: well, it wasn't all women. The great Stanley Way in Newcastle started off many years ago and I used to go and work with him, and he would tell me of the early days when he had been trained by Ruth Graham, who had worked with George Papanicolaou.[28] Way came back to Gateshead and to Newcastle in the late 1950s–early 1960s and for many years used to do all the work to prepare the

---

[25] A later handbook was Bloch *et al.* (eds) (1995).

[26] Professor Dulcie Coleman wrote: 'My first appointment was at the Hillingdon Hospital, London. Pathology was located in the former sitting room of an old Victorian house on the hospital site. I think the building has been torn down now.' Letter to Mrs Lois Reynolds, 8 October 2009.

[27] For details of the current MSc in clinical cytology, see www1.imperial.ac.uk/medicine/teaching/shortcourses/teaching/clinicalcytology/ (visited 23 June 2009).

[28] See, for example, Way (1963); Stening (1950). Dr James Andrew reflected that Mr Way described colposcopy as 'the biggest confidence trick ever perpetrated in the name of gynaecology', although Newcastle later acquired a colposcope (Andrew (1975): 4).

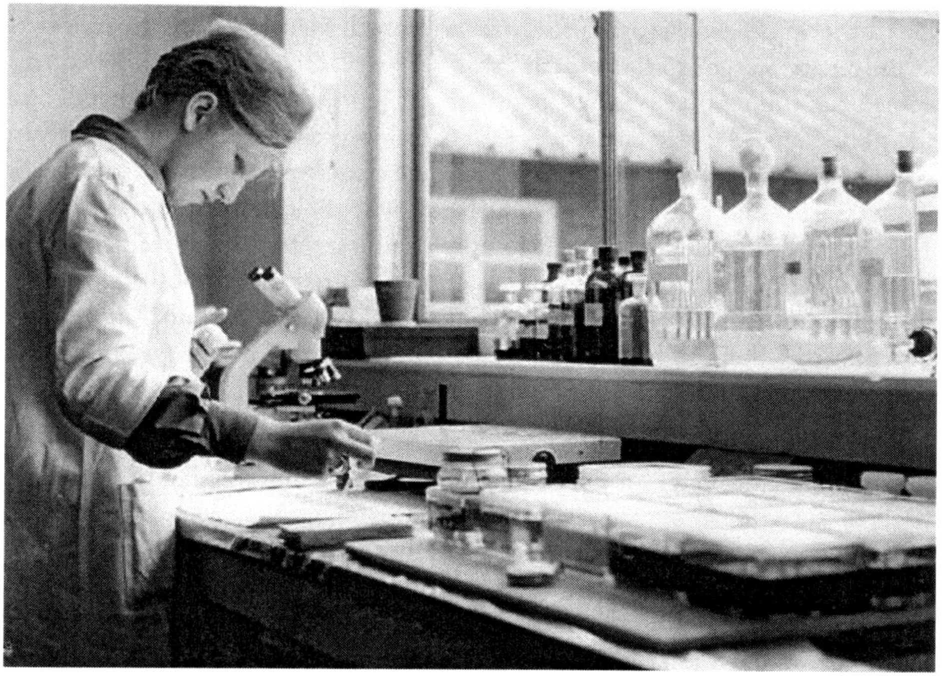

Figure 2: Mrs Marilyn Symonds, cytology laboratory, Stoke Mandeville Hospital, Aylesbury, 1964.

slides and read them himself. One day he told me this story of how it came to be that there was a five-year screening interval – the Government used to say it was five years – and he said, 'Well, they asked me one day down to a meeting and they said how many years do you think there should be for an interval?' and he said: 'Well, I really didn't know, there was no evidence, so I thought five-yearly was a reasonable target.'[29] He would still read his own cytology until he retired; he was one of the originators.

Mackenzie: May I say that the other mentor I must not forget is Elizabeth Macgregor in Aberdeen [Figure 1].[30] She was formative as far as screening in this country was concerned, and when you think she was at the top of Great Britain – we in Scotland are still part of GB, I presume, tucked away up there – and her work was exemplary, proper screening, properly managed. It took the rest of the UK about 30 years to catch up with her.

---

[29] Glucksmann *et al.* (1964) suggested that mortality increased between the fifth and tenth years of follow-up of patients treated between 1952 and 1962 (page 200); Way (1954, 1962, 1969); Guthrie *et al.* (1981). See also DHSS, Committee on Gynaecological Cytology (1981).

[30] See also notes 5, 38, 163, 164 and 174; Figure 1, page 9.

Dr Catherine Pike: I was going to say that Elizabeth Macgregor was my colleague at university, we got to know each other very well. I got into cytology when I came back from Africa, where I had been for ten years with my husband, and the phone rang one day and it was Elizabeth Macgregor saying: 'What are you going to do? What about doing cytology?' The next thing was that I arrived at St Thomas' Hospital with Professor John Tighe, who took an interest in cytology.[31] I was trained there, but also went to other training sessions and trained others as well.[32] In a very busy south London area, we were taught from the word go to follow up women with abnormal smears, and that it was most important; you didn't let them slide through the system. We started a card system, always following up women with abnormal smears, making sure that they were seen by a gynaecologist for assessment and treatment.

Dr Amanda Herbert: Can I say something further about Stanley Way, because back in those days it was very often gynaecologists who were encouraging screening, whereas pathologists were woefully apathetic about it. When he was the chairman of the BSCC, he wrote a brilliant letter in the *BMJ*, saying how hopeless Kenneth Robinson's proposal was for setting up the 1967 programme, largely because it wasn't adequately funded. He went through the press release bit by bit, in a beautifully written letter, pointing out that it wasn't going to work if it wasn't properly funded – and if cytologists didn't have long enough to train.[33] Nearly 20 years later the *Lancet* editorial, 'Death by incompetence' fulfilled his prediction.[34]

McCluggage: I am going to move to a related topic, that is, who became a cytologist and why, and ask Dr Gray, because this leads on very nicely from what we have just been talking about.

Dr Winifred Gray: I think a lot has already been said by previous speakers about their own experience in this particular area. Throughout the 1960s women

---

[31] See, for example, Tighe (1961); Fruin and Tighe (1967).

[32] Dr Catherine Pike wrote: 'I received additional training at the Royal Free Hospital with Dr Chandra Grubb in a few informal sessions, as far as I remember. I always attended the well-organized workshops at the annual scientific meetings of the BSCC, at first relating to gynaecological cytology but soon covering all aspects of non-cervical cytology.' Note on draft transcript, 29 August 2009. For a list of scientific meetings and the papers given, see BSCC (1983).

[33] Mr Kenneth Robinson's press conference on 21 October 1966 was reported in the *BMJ* (Anon. (1966)); Way's ripost appeared the following February (Way (1967)). See also Glossary, pages 149–50. For later details of screening programme, see Spratley (1990).

[34] Anon. (1985).

doctors needing part-time work for domestic reasons were often responsible for the reporting of abnormal smears. Some worked within a gynaecology department, where an individual gynaecologist had a special interest in the work.[35] Others became involved at the time of establishing the BSCC in 1961, as already mentioned, such as Dr Arthur Spriggs, who was a haematologist originally. He was responsible for gynaecological and non-gynaecological cytology in Oxford and played a significant part in attempts at automating the screening of cervical smears.[36] He also investigated the impact of the failure to follow up abnormal smears, with an elaborate tracing of women across the country whom his laboratory had found to have abnormal smears, but who hadn't returned for treatment.[37]

Another factor that hasn't come into the discussion so far is the role of the College of Pathologists in the training of histopathologists in cytology, and encouraging them to take the area of gynaecological cytology seriously. It was really completely separate from histology in the department in Oxford where I worked. It was referred to as the 'dregs' by those who weren't involved at all, and it was certainly not looked upon as a very prestigious area to be working in as a histopathologist. I think the college did eventually acknowledge that training was required, that an examination in cytology should be included in the college exams. Certainly, when I took the MRCPath final in 1971, cytology was beginning to be included. I think when I had my finals viva, the two examiners were more nervous than I was, because here was this cytopathologist and they didn't quite know what on earth to ask me. They got their own back in the afternoon by giving me an amputated penis for a histological specimen.

Gradually, through the 1970s and 1980s, the college has become more and more aware of the need to have a proper qualification that involves cytology and particularly gynaecological cytology, along with histology. It's interesting that

---

[35] Dr Winifred Gray wrote: 'I was one of the first to have a full training in pathology at the Radcliffe Infirmary, starting in 1969, under the married women's retraining scheme which was started by Dr Rosemary Rue, public health consultant in the Oxford NHS administration. This scheme enabled women with family commitments to have a part-time training post in a teaching hospital. It led to several other women qualifying for consultant posts where before they remained as clinical or medical assistants.' Letter to Mrs Lois Reynolds, 12 September 2009. See Rue (1967); see also Colville and Wenban (1972); Duncan (ed.) (1992); Anon. (1968).

[36] For details of Dr Arthur Spriggs' work, see note 19, Appendix 2 and his Biographical note on pages 140–1.

[37] Kinlen and Spriggs (1978); Spriggs and Boddington (1980). Dr Winifred Gray wrote: 'This study provided convincing evidence of the ability of cervical cytology to prevent the development of cervical cancer.' Note on draft transcript, 26 August 2009.

in 1998, at an international meeting held in Oxford, the then president of the college apologized for the lack of support that had been given to proper training, particularly in cervical cytology, so I do think that has now been addressed.[38]

McCluggage: Certainly, cervical cytology is much more important now. The people who started off doing cervical cytology, were they mainly specializing in that, or were they also doing non-gynaecological cytology and histopathology?

Gray: No, it was usually both. With the sub-specialization that is now so prevalent, some pathologists are specializing solely in gynaecological cytology and histology. But in most district general hospitals, pathologists still have to be responsible for all aspects of cytology. That's what I understand.

Jenkins: If I can join in here? When I was training in histopathology, cervical cytology was certainly despised in some of the institutions in the 1970s where I was trained and in others there was great enthusiasm. Catherine Pike and John Tighe were probably the people who trained me most in cytology at St Thomas', but other institutions really didn't take it seriously at all. I think the examination (MRCPath) was simply six slides that were carefully selected, so that they were either normal or cancerous. It was very much a token effort.

> [Professor Valerie Beral raised the question of international perspective, as it wasn't clear from the discussion whether the meeting was concerned solely with the cervical screening programme in the UK or elsewhere. She suggested that Jocelyn Chamberlain, Tony Miller and others could discuss what is going on in Scandinavia, British Columbia and elsewhere.

---

[38] Dr Margaret Wolfendale wrote: 'The part played by the BSCC was inadvertently omitted in the Witness Seminar. Following the first International Meeting on Cytology in 1961 held in Vienna, a meeting was convened by a small number of enthusiasts who were already practising cytology and the BSCC was founded to promote the growth and development of clinical cytology in the UK. It proceeded to play a crucial role in promoting cervical screening by bringing together individuals struggling in comparative isolation, by sharing scientific information at their annual meetings, laying down standards of practice, encouraging the setting up of training schools and setting up a "certificate of competence" for screeners, headed by Michael Boddington. From the start there was a small non-medical membership which was expanded to 10 per cent, then 20 per cent, an innovative move that was looked down on by many medical colleagues in other specialties. In further recognition of the vital need for continuing education of the whole of the laboratory team, the setting up of regional societies was supported and by 1973 the whole of the country was covered by affiliated societies holding regular scientific meetings. A prime example of an initiative to raise standards was the publication in 1981 of a guide, *Taking Uterine Cervical Smears* (Macgregor (1981)), the first 10 000 copies rapidly sold out. A new second edition was published in 1989 (revised edition 1995) accompanied by a video, sales of which were also extremely successful.' Note on draft transcript, 26 November 2008. The BSCC Report for 1961–83 notes that 15 000 copies were initially sold (BSCC (1983): 14).

She asked whether it was from these programmes that people in the UK began to understand how screening worked.]

Professor Jocelyn Chamberlain: During the same period, in Sweden and Finland and to a lesser extent in Denmark, but not Norway, screening was introduced as a coordinated public health programme, aiming to reach the whole eligible population.[39] Elizabeth Macgregor in Aberdeen, as far as I know was the only person in Britain who really succeeded in doing that prior to the re-organization of the UK screening programme in the late 1980s.[40] There's very convincing and positive evidence when you compare the incidence and mortality rates of invasive cervical cancer in Sweden and Finland with those in Norway, where there was no organized screening, during the 1970s, the rates come straight down in the two countries that were doing it in a systemic, organized way.[41] Their eligibility criteria were such that to be invited to be screened a woman should, I think, be aged between 25 and 69, and should not have had a normal test within the previous five years – between 70 per cent and 80 per cent of women accepted their invitations.

Professor Anthony Miller: I want to thank the organizers for bringing me here. I have spent all my life in terms of cervical screening in Canada and I happen to be visiting at the moment, although the first part of my life was spent in the UK. In fact I was in the Medical Research Council (MRC) tuberculosis research unit in 1970 – to link up with something that was said earlier – when, as I was going to a conference in New York, I was invited to look at an automated cytology set-up there. I did and came back to report to the MRC and also to O A N Husain – normally known as Nasseem – with whom I discussed this, although they didn't think that particular mechanism worked.[42]

---

[39] Professor Jocelyn Chamberlain wrote: 'In the 1960s and 1970s, as we have seen, cervical screening developed here in a haphazard way, with decisions on who should be screened and how often, being taken on the whim of individual clinicians working without guidance, and the cytology laboratories responding as best they could to this uncoordinated demand.' Note on draft transcript, 31 July 2008. See, for example, Hakama (1982).

[40] Macgregor *et al.* (1971); for a discussion of the data, see Wilson *et al.* (1971). For background of the policy changes concerning cervical screening, see note 155; Glossary, pages 148–51.

[41] IARC Working Group on evaluation of cervical cancer screening programmes (1986). See also Hill and Adelstein (1967).

[42] A combined research group of Drs N Jankey, H Ferreira, C B Cameron and O A N Husain (Chelsea Hospital for Women, Royal Marsden and St Stephen's Hospital, Chelsea) gave a preliminary account of the use of the Coulter counter in cancer screening at the fourth annual scientific meeting of the British Society for Clinical Cytology in October 1965 (Anon (1965)); see also pages 90–1.

A bit more history, because people haven't given much history: in terms of the perception internationally over cervical cytology, many of you will know the paper of H S Ahluwalia and Sir Richard Doll, which effectively looked at the decline in cervical cancer mortality in a number of countries, including Canada, and concluded that cervical screening was not working.[43] In my MRC links, before I went to the National Cancer Institute of Canada, I used to interact with Archie Cochrane, and Archie was very much of the belief that it didn't work and he told me that I had to go to Canada to show that it didn't work.[44] When I went to Canada, the National Cancer Institute of Canada, together with the American Cancer Society, had started funding an evaluation of the British Columbia programme at that time. The British Columbia programme was established in 1949 by Herb Fidler, a pathologist, who brought David Boyes into his programme. Boyes, originally a family physician who trained as a pathologist and a gynaecologist, became a leader in Canada in terms of cervical cancer screening. They kept meticulous records. So when a group of us, including George Knox from Birmingham, started evaluating these records at the beginning of the 1970s, it became clear that there was a good resource for evaluating the natural history of cervical cancer, and that resource was eventually published.[45] The data were published and incorporated into something that Professor Nicholas Day was doing – unfortunately he can't be here today – who was working in the International Agency for Research on Cancer (IARC) in Lyons at that time in the mid-1980s. He evaluated the data in terms of models, and demonstrated that you didn't have to screen annually, that you got almost the maximum benefit by three-yearly or five-yearly screening, and, of course, this has been replicated subsequently.[46] Perhaps Peter Sasieni will talk about some of his studies in the UK.

We were challenged nationally in Canada to try to demonstrate that screening worked, and we set up a study to evaluate the extent to which mortality had

---

[43] Ahluwalia and Doll (1968).

[44] Dr Archie Cochrane wrote: 'Apart from the immunization programme the record of the NHS is patchy. There are sins of omission and commission. Of the latter the introduction of the programme of cervical smears in the hope of preventing carcinoma of the cervix is the saddest. It illustrates so clearly the consequences of assuming a hypothesis is correct, and translating the consequences into routine clinical practice before testing it by an RCT.' Cochrane (1972): 26–7. See also note 162.

[45] Boyes *et al.* (1982); see also Shun-Zhang *et al.* (1982). For questions arising from the natural history of carcinoma *in situ,* see Knox (1966).

[46] Hakama *et al.* (eds) (1986).

fallen in different parts of the country.[47] We had to use cancer of the uterus because there was a changing certification of whether you certify as cancer of the cervix specifically or the uterus unspecified, so we took the whole of uterine cancer, did a correlation analysis, and it was extremely clear: no matter what factors you took into consideration, the areas which had the greatest intensity of screening had the greatest reduction in mortality. This was very influential for convincing people in Canada that this worked. It was the Walton Committee in 1976 that built on that.[48] Eventually I think the Americans were persuaded, and even Archie Cochrane was eventually persuaded that it worked.

One last point relates to the fact that very much later, through Jan Pontén, who was chairman of the Swedish Cancer Society, we were able to evaluate historical records in the Karolinska Institute. It became very clear that the introduction of radiotherapy, basically radium therapy, had a major impact on mortality from cancer of the cervix in Sweden before screening came in.[49] So Richard Doll (Figure 3, top row, right) in many respects was right, there was a reduction going on, largely because of improvements in treatment, but that had come to an end, and then when screening came in and people began to find precursors and incidence fell, then mortality fell not long after. So history sometimes is quite right.

Professor Jack Cuzick: I remember – I think, very much based on George Knox's wonderful editorial 'Death by incompetence'[50] – in 1973 we set up the Imperial Cancer Research Fund (ICRF) coordinating committee on cervical screening,[51] and very much with Husain's strong leadership, managed to put together some statements about what was needed, and the fact that, although Nick Day had shown clearly that screening could reduce mortality, it wasn't happening in the UK at that time.[52] We published a position paper in the *BMJ* in 1985 and then subsequently another paper, which I think was very much the basis of the

---

[47] Miller *et al.* (1976).

[48] See, for example, Walton *et al.* (1976, 1982); Kassirer (1980).

[49] Pontén *et al.* (1995).

[50] Anon (1985).

[51] ICRF, Coordinating Committee on cervical screening (1984). Members of the committee were: Walter Bodmer, Jocelyn Chamberlain, Gary Cook, Jack Cuzick (secretary), Gerald Draper, Stephen Erskine, Hugh Fisher, Rod Griffiths, David Haran, Christine Havelock, O A N Husain, E G Knox, Ann McPherson, Alwyn Smith, Arthur Spriggs, David Innes Williams (chair) and Margaret Wolfendale.

[52] IARC Working Group on evaluation of cervical cancer screening programmes (1986).

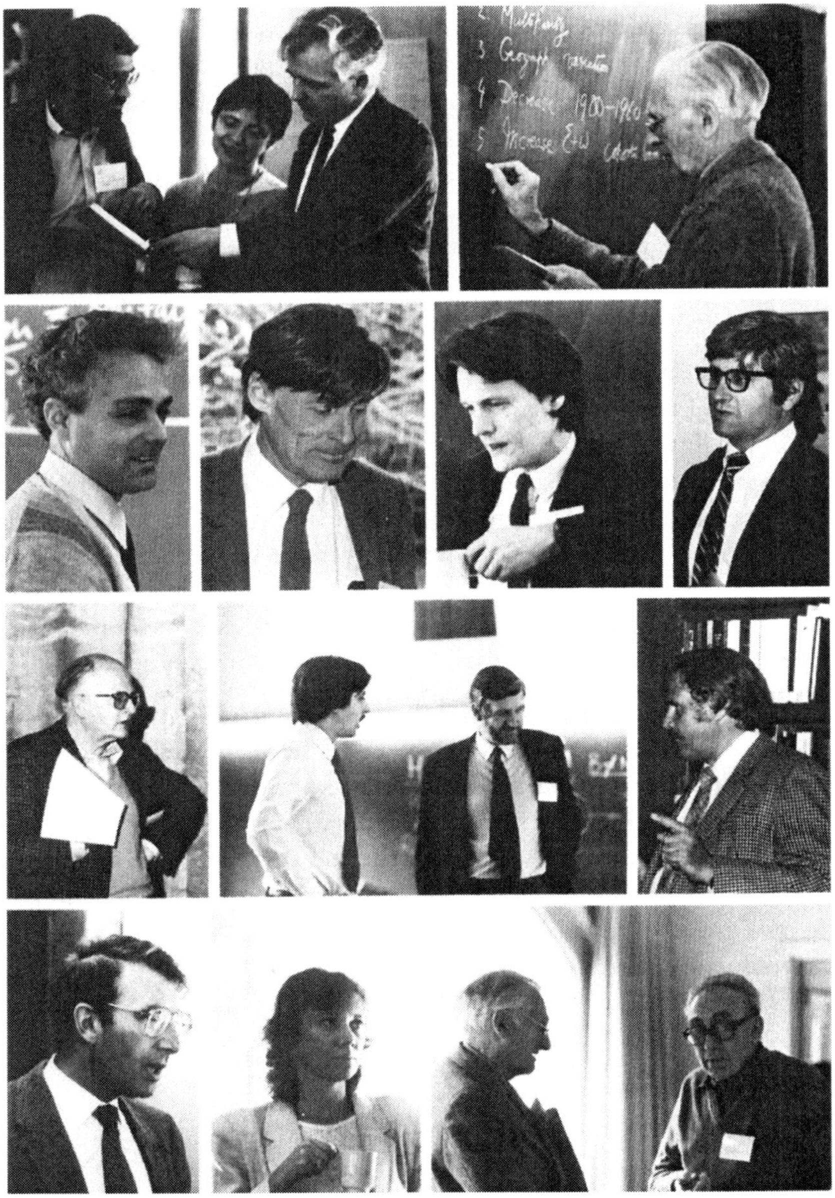

Figure 3: Contributors to the 1985 Banbury Center conference on 'The origins of female genital cancer'.
L to R from top row: J R Schlehofer, Elke-Ingrid Grussendorf-Conen, Harald zur Hausen, Richard Doll; row 2: Thomas Broker, J Cairns, Richard Peto, P M Howley; row 3: Erich Burghardt; Attila Lörincz, Martin Vessey, Richard Reid; bottom row: Albert Singer, Louise Brinton, Richard Doll, Leopold Koss. (Peto and zur Hausen (eds) (1986): frontispiece).

national programme that was set up here, identifying the requirements for that national programme and I think that's an important landmark as well.[53]

McCluggage: I think we are going to talk more about this later. We are going to move on now to something we have already touched on, life and interactions in a cervical screening laboratory.

Mrs Marilyn Symonds: I am speaking from the cytotechnology angle, from the technicians' side. I also started in cytology a very long time ago with Dr Margaret Wolfendale in 1963. It was absolutely unheard of for student medical laboratory technicians to be employed solely in a cytology laboratory, because there were no formal qualifications to become associates and fellows of what is now the Institute of Biomedical Science (IBMS).[54] So you had to qualify along the histology route and, just to let you know, that the cytology question in my histology final was to take a buccal smear (a sample of cells from inside of the cheek) from myself and stain it, using a Papanicolaou technique. I don't think that stood me in very good stead to actually be able to diagnose abnormalities in cervical smears.

I heard from all of you pioneers in cervical cytology that very soon you wanted to pass over all that boring screening stuff to some technical people. To start with, the type of people who worked in a cytology department technically were histology technicians, mainly female again, except for one very well-known exception, Dennis Williams, who I am sorry is not here to support me today. He started with the Birmingham crew and has done an enormous amount of work to help recognize the important role of the non-medical person working in cytology. To start with, we had people who were formally training to be laboratory technicians and then I think it was probably in the 1970s that we took on a group of women, mainly part-time, who became cytoscreeners. They were different to the people who were qualified with the IBMS; they didn't have any formal qualifications, and they were often derided and called shopping-bag screeners, but they were absolutely fantastic at what they did. They were able to sit down quietly and concentrate and look at every cell that was being passed under the microscope, and I can say that that group of women now are nearly all retired, and it's extremely difficult to replace them. The IBMS now think that

---

[53] Cuzick *et al.* (1998); Cuzick and Sasieni (2001).

[54] For a history of the Institute, see www.ibms.org/index.cfm?method=science.history_zone&subpage=IBMS_history (visited 13 August 2009).

we should have biomedical scientists with degrees, and formal qualifications in cytology, but I can honestly say that on the whole they are not nearly as good at screening as those women from the 1960s and 1970s.

One of the most exciting things for me was the interaction, together with my medical colleagues, with the pathologists, and also with the GPs, because we were talking about setting up a screening programme in Aylesbury, Dr Margaret Wolfendale, myself, and a couple of other people. We set up a screening programme based on the electoral roll, so we wrote out invitation cards, little postcards, and we went round the villages in the rural district of Aylesbury, and delivered these personally ourselves to try to encourage the women to come to clinics and have their smears done. Then there were a few very, very enthusiastic GPs who were supporting us and they used to come in, deliver the smears they had taken, and meet us in the laboratory and we felt part of this wider team. And I think this is what cytology still is, within pathology medicine, that we all know our GPs, we have a lot of interaction with the practice nurses who now take all the smears, and we are quite different from the other laboratories.

Jenkins: One of the questions that has always intrigued me was what made cytoscreeners, the women who weren't trained as technicians, become cytoscreeners, because as you say it is a tremendously difficult job, it involves enormous patience and is something that a lot of us couldn't do. Why did people take up this job?

Symonds: One of the things was that we offered them part-time working, so it fitted in very well with the ethos of our medical pathologists. They were mainly married women with children, who wanted an interesting job to fit around their home commitments. A lot of them had had some scientific background of working within perhaps research, before they had their children, or perhaps had worked in school laboratories.

Coleman: I wanted to add one thing that I think is not always appreciated and which we found – because I was very much involved in teaching – that you think of screening as being very dreary and routine. In fact every smear is different and is a challenge, and I think only screeners, people who do it every day, really appreciate that, and I think that's what keeps me going.

Wolfendale: We are really talking about the backbone of the cytology laboratory, where these were almost all married screeners who worked part-time – they were paid peanuts, absolute peanuts – and the only way that we managed to keep them was making it teamwork, making them feel really worthwhile and wanted, and they felt that it was something interesting that they could do to get away from their family routines.[55] I think, it was an almost pastoral care that we gave, supporting each other through all sorts of troubles. Last year I was invited back, ten years after I had retired, and there were really a large number of the people who had worked during the 40 years that the laboratory had been going and had come back because it was a team effort. And I am sure many, many other people in laboratories would say the same.

McCluggage: I have always heard anecdotally that it is very difficult to get people to go into screening. Is it still difficult? And are the problems getting better or worse?

Miller: I would like to make the comment that Dave Boyes in British Columbia went out of his way to find people who couldn't find jobs elsewhere – some of them, in fact, were in wheelchairs, were paraplegic – and there were many men who fell into that category employed in his very large laboratory that served the whole of the province. So it is sometimes possible, if you look, to find people who really need employment and are prepared to spend the time.

Symonds: I think the answer to the question whether it is easy to recruit staff now is 'no', it's impossible. Everybody who has worked in cytology labs for many years is retiring, the people who are replacing them are not prepared to sit down quietly in the same way, and I think there are so many more demands on them. Especially in the south of England, it's virtually impossible to recruit staff. So I would say thank goodness for liquid-based cytology (LBC). I know that is not what we are talking about today, but with LBC comes the possibility of automation, which will help reduce the staffing crisis.[56]

Herbert: We don't find it impossible to recruit staff, especially now we have biomedical scientists (BMS), who don't only do cervical cytology. They have quite a lot of other things to do and cytology screening is part of the general BMS qualification.[57] We haven't employed cytology screeners as such for some

---

[55] Wolfendale (1991).

[56] Mrs Marilyn Symonds wrote: 'My hospital, Stoke Mandeville, was involved in a five-site research project in 1996 comparing conventional screening to the PAPNET automatic screening method. The outcome was that cytoscreeners were as effective at detection of abnormalities as the machines. Twelve years later, trials using automated assisted screening are still taking place.' Note on draft transcript, 28 August 2008.

[57] See 'Qualifications and training for non-medical laboratory staff in the UK cervical screening programmes' (January 2000) at www.cancerscreening.nhs.uk/cervical/publications/nhscsp12.pdf (visited 30 April 2009).

time and we seem to have been able to recruit people reasonably easily in London. We have had times when it was difficult, but not impossible.

McCluggage: We will move on to another very important subject: given the expansion in cervical screening, obviously colposcopy has increased as well.

Duncan: Yesterday I went into the old byre and dug out stuff that had been in a wheelbarrow since I retired at the end of March 2007. I found something I thought was quite interesting; it was published in an obscure thing called *Colposcopy and Gynaecological Laser Surgery*, published in 1987, and it was my observations as the then president of the British Society for Colposcopy and Cervical Pathology (BSCCP).[58] You have asked me specifically to look at the 1980s, rather than the 1970s when it all began. I was reflecting, if you like, following the annual meeting of the BSCCP. The BSCCP really was established in the 1970s. Albert Singer was one of the original protagonists in 1972 when the society was founded. The founding trio, Joe Jordan, Albert Singer and Archie Crompton – that was it – met in 1972. I was training in the US at the time, came back in 1974 and the society was formed in 1975.[59] From humble beginnings, it grew in leaps and bounds, and by 1987 the membership was over 500. We used to meet annually. The BSCCP met twice a year, once on our own, and once with the BSCC and then we separated because there was more to talk about. The first problem that I was addressing in this publication was who should be undergoing colposcopic examination.[60] We had found out that the smears themselves did not actually tell you what the underlying problem was. Yes, high-grade smears tended to indicate high-grade cervical intraepithelial neoplasia (CIN) – as we were calling it then – and low-grade smears tended to indicate low-grade lesions. However, when the patient with a low-grade smear was examined with a colposcope, she often had a high-grade lesion, usually, much smaller, but a high-grade lesion was visible also. So it was a question of should we be seeing women with originally positive smears? Suspicious smears? These were the class IVs and the IIIs.[61] But then the class II smears and mild atypia, should we be seeing them? What we were saying at that time was that there seemed to be justification for doing it, but it

---

[58] Duncan (1987); see also note 59.

[59] For the history of the BSCCP, see www.bsccp.org.uk/index.asp?PageID=15 (visited 13 August 2009).

[60] Duncan (ed.) (1992). See also Anon (1968).

[61] These classes refer to the guidelines for the interpretation of smears proposed by Papanicolaou. See Koss and Melamed (2006).

could increase our workload dramatically, and until the supply met the demand, patients would have to be seen on a priority basis. The question was then whether you should do follow-up colposcopy, or reserve your colposcopy for the primary problem. And then who should be carrying out colposcopy? It's very much like the cytologists. At that time the vice-president of the BSCCP was a pathologist, so he wasn't a gynaecologist, and at the annual scientific meeting that year, a general practitioner colposcopist addressed us in Aviemore, Scotland, on how she was operating a successful practice here in London. Then we were discussing what treatment was appropriate. What we agreed in the end, after quite a bit of work, was that it didn't matter whether you treated them with local destruction using extremes of heat or cold, or whether you used some method of excision, these had all been shown to be equally effective. As long as you didn't overdo the cervical treatment, then there was no injury to future cervical function. We all agreed to disagree, if you like, and found all methods were acceptable. We had also encountered *in situ* adenocarcinoma of the cervix. This was something that had come out of cytology, and we were wondering exactly what we should be doing with that. What we had also found was that women who had vulvar warts, about 30 per cent of them were harbouring CIN as well, and so the question arose should women with vulvar warts actually be seen, and should their partners who had penile warts, should they be examined colposcopically as a routine? And should they be treated as well? So these were the things that were perplexing us, and the last paragraph of this publication said:

> I have attempted to highlight the main problems facing us. There are, of course, many others, from the particular (eg, what is the true significance of HPV16?) to the more general (eg, what public health measures are necessary to stem the flood of CIN?). We live in a world where the fear of pregnancy has been removed by the contraceptive pill, where the protective effect of the sheath against sexually transmitted infection has been lost due to the fall in popularity of barrier methods. Sexual liberty and gratification are regularly portrayed on television and used unashamedly by the advertising industry. It should come as little surprise to us that we are seeing more and more cases of CIN just as we are seeing more genital warts, chlamydia and more cases of unwanted pregnancy. It is ironic that it may take something like the government education programme engendered by a fear of an AIDS epidemic to alter public opinion and sexual practice in such a way as to provide primary prevention of invasive cervical cancer.[62]

---

[62] Duncan (1987).

I had attempted to highlight the main problems facing us, there were, of course, many others: from the particular, for example, what is the true significance of HPV16, to the more general, such as whether public health measures were necessary to stem the flood of CIN.[63] I said that perhaps the government education programme as then being applied to the AIDS epidemic might be beneficial to us, but meanwhile the BSCCP would continue to have its say in the setting and maintaining of standards for the present-day colposcopists and the continued quest for tomorrow's knowledge. And that's really carried on in the same way since then. So that was the 1980s.

McCluggage: Anybody else want to comment on that?

Coleman: I can recall one important meeting, I think it was called the Intercollegiate Working Party on cervical cytology screening, which I think Albert Singer drew together and perhaps he could comment on that.[64] That was 1988 and I remember the results of that meeting were published in the *BMJ* and that seemed to transform cytology from the desperate confused situation into a more directive programme, and laid the foundation I thought, for what, in my view, is the first-class cervical screening programme that we have today.[65] Perhaps Albert could comment on that.

Mr Patrick Walker: I'm from the Royal Free Hospital, London. I started working with Albert Singer in 1981 as a research fellow interested in HPV. To throw a little bit of light on a question that has never really been fully understood: why was colposcopy very slow to get off the ground in the UK? Hans Hinselmann's first paper was in October 1925 and from then on it became reasonably popular on the mainland continent of Europe.[66] The Gynaecological Visiting Society of Great Britain and Ireland (GVS) was founded by Blair-Bell in 1911, who later went on to found the Royal College of Obstetricians and

---

[63] Duncan (ed.) (1997).

[64] Dr Ian Duncan wrote: 'It was not Albert Singer who was the chairman, but Frank Sharp from the Royal College of Obstetricians and Gynaecologists.' Note on transcript, 2 September 2008. The brief was to look at the clinical aspects of cervical cytopathology screening programme in the UK, see Royal College of Obstetricians and Gynecologists, Royal College of Pathologists, Royal College of General Practitioners and Faculty of Community Medicine, Intercollegiate Working Party (1987).

[65] Havelock *et al.* (1988).

[66] Hinselmann (1925); for the early history, see O'Dowd and Philipp (1994): 30–1; 550–1; 531–4; 543–70; 640–1.

Gynaecologists.[67] The society was a travelling group; they were the elite travelling group of the professors from the British medical schools and they travelled in 1937 to Berlin, stopping off on the way in Hamburg. They were greeted by Professor Hinselmann who took them to his home for tea and then the following day took them to his colposcopy unit in Altona, the hospital where he practised colposcopy. These were difficult times in Europe and it is alleged that Hinselmann – I think it is probably true – was quite a prominent member of the National Socialist Party at the time. What the GVS used to do was to assess surgical procedures, see how to do things slightly differently, and as the convenor of the GVS at the moment, I have the records going back to that meeting. One of the operations that they saw was a sterilization at a time that forced sterilizations were allowed in Germany. So when they came back from Germany, there was no enthusiasm for either Hinselmann or his technique, although Fletcher Shaw arranged for one colposcope to be delivered to the UK, and Dr James Andrew found one in the outpatients at Bart's in the 1950s. By then Andrew was running a monthly colposcopy clinic there through the 1960s.[68]

A personal remembrance: when I was a medical student at Bart's in 1972, Gordon Bourne was the senior gynaecologist and there was an afternoon tutorial. We were all trying to rush off to the bar or somewhere else, and he said: 'No, please stay behind. There's a very nice man called Dr James Andrew who is coming to talk to you about a German instrument called a colposcope, which none of us feels has any value, but he's an awfully nice man, why don't you stay and listen to him'. And I did and I didn't know then that later on in my life it would mean something. I think that until Albert Singer came from Coppleson's unit, Joe Jordan had been with Per Kolstad and Archie Crompton with Professor Ernst Navratil, they came together to form the British Colposcopy Group in 1972, the previous hiatus actually had something of a medico–political dimension.[69]

---

[67] Shaw (1950, 1954a and b). Sir William Fletcher Shaw was the first honorary secretary of the Royal College of Obstetricians and Gynaecologists in 1929, later president (1938–43).

[68] Dr James Andrew described his first Zeiss colposcope and setting up his regular colposcopy clinic at Bart's in 1954 in a paper, 'British colposcopy before the 1960s' (Andrew (1975)). A copy of the paper will be deposited along with other records of the meeting in archives and manuscripts, Wellcome Library, London, in GC/253. See also Jordan (1975); Burghardt *et al.* (eds) (1978).

[69] See also Kolstad (1970).

Herbert: One of the things that colposcopy did for cytology in the 1980s was to focus laboratories on quality control, which greatly improved when the real programme started in 1988. Colposcopists were seeing patients with borderline smears and persistent mild abnormalities and finding they had CIN3. Obviously not all of them, but it made cytologists focus on quality control.

The other thing – and Jocelyn Chamberlain is here – was her excellent article on the reasons why screening may fail to prevent cancer, which was very important.[70] Among those reasons were false negative cytology, low-grade abnormalities that were high-grade on review, and failure to follow up after treatment.[71] When colposcopists were seeing women with what were thought to be minor abnormalities on cytology, it became a bit of a bone of contention between pathologists and cytologists. I think that was one of the reasons why the two organizations split and held different meetings.[72]

Duncan: Dulcie was speaking about this Intercollegiate Working Party, which Albert has passed on to me, because I don't think Albert was involved. It was under the chairmanship of Frank Sharp, who along with myself, represented the Royal College of Obstetricians and Gynaecologists. Dr D M D Evans and Professor Harold Fox represented the Royal College of Pathologists; Dr P B Havelock and Dr Ann McPherson from the Royal College of General Practitioners; and Dr Jocelyn Chamberlain and Professor Alwyn Smith from the Faculty of Community Medicine.[73] What it did was to publish a report in November 1987 and it actually set out who should have smears, how often and when, putting together what was happening in the Department of Health in Scotland, which had issued a statement,[74] and the DHS which had also issued

---

[70] Chamberlain (1986).

[71] See, for example, Cuzick *et al.* (1994).

[72] Dr Amanda Herbert wrote: 'The BSCCP met during the BSCC annual meeting until 1982 and I think not thereafter.' Note on draft transcript, 23 July 2009.

[73] Although the BSCC were not officially represented on the Intercollegiate Working Party, the society provided two appendices to the *Report* (RCOG *et al.* (1987)): 'Recommended code of practice for laboratories providing a cytopathology service' and 'Terminology in gynaecological cytopathology, report of the working party of the BSCC', the members of which were D M D Evans (chairman), E A Hudson (secretary), C L Brown, M M Boddington, H E Hughes, E F Mackenzie and T Marshall, and had been published in the *Journal of Clinical Pathology* (Evans *et al.* (1986)).

[74] Scottish Health Service Planning Council, Scientific Services Advisory Group, Subcommittee on Histopathology (1977). See Glossary, pages 150–1.

a statement.[75] And that led one year later to the founding of the NHS Cervical Screening Programme national coordinating network which was basically the 14 English health regions, the three Celtic nations, and the private sector (the big 18).[76] And, up until devolution, then it worked and produced a series of documents and Amanda Herbert edited some, I edited some, Catherine Pike did some as well. So that really got us all together, and it became a quality-assured service with quality control and fail-safe mechanisms and all of that. That is where Euphemia McGoogan came in, the missing link, the Edinburgh one, who was, if you like, a second-generation cytologist, and then she took a lead role as well.[77]

McCluggage: I think we will probably touch on this later on, but we are going to move on to the discovery of the HPV and the development of HPV research. Albert Singer is going to make a few brief comments about the unknown male factor.

Singer: In four minutes. It is certainly a privilege and rather humbling after 40 years to go back and look at – as you say – the unknown male factor, and especially working with so many colleagues after all those years. I started off in the mid-1960s, in Sydney, Australia, joining up with Professor Malcolm Coppleson who has already been mentioned – he was a colposcopist and a gynaecological oncologist – and Bevan Reid who was a cell biologist, a brilliant scientist; and in the early 1960s they were studying the process of squamous metaplasia, the process by which columnar epithelium changes to squamal and during that time the observation was made that sperm heads were found in the regenerating cells. They believed that the stromal cells underneath the epithelium were the progenitor cells of the new squamous epithelium, and they absorbed the sperm DNA. That culminated in the classic pictures by Bevan Reid in the *Lancet* of a sperm fragment in a cervical cell.[78] I was taken on as a research fellow in 1966,

---

[75] Department of Health and Social Security (DHSS) (1986a), later consolidated as DHSS (1988). It recommended that all women between the ages of 20 and 64 should be invited for screening within five years of 31 March 1988. For details of the narrowing of the age range in 2004, see note 155.

[76] Dr J A Muir Gray, as chairman of the National Coordinating Network (NCN), convened a group of regional contacts and professional associations in cervical cancer screening about their training and educational needs. The resulting report, 'Education and training needs of programme managers' was published in 1989 and is no longer in print. See www.cancerscreening.nhs.uk/cervical/publications/pm-01.html (visited 3 September 2009).

[77] See Biographical notes, pages 137–8.

[78] Reid (1964); see also Coppleson and Reid (1969); Singer and Reid (1976).

and the only other research fellow was my good friend Margaret Stanley, but she was 700 miles away in Adelaide. Both of us worked on the cervix and my first task was to imitate squamous metaplasia.

What I did was to take women who were down for cervical cauterization, which destroyed the cervical epithelium and then watched the regeneration. When they would say to us: 'Can I go with my husband or partner?' we said to them, 'That's all right', because the reason was to see if we could imitate Bevan Reid's original findings, and sure enough, in many of the women the regenerating cervical cells (we published this in publications in 1967) showed that sperm was taken up. And that led us to the concept that maybe it was the sperm DNA mixing with the endogenous DNA. But for all the tissue culture work we could not go much further with it. I then left in 1970 to come here; Reid continued. He moved away from DNA, worked mainly on basic proteins protamine and histones in sperm, and in 1978, in a rather contentious and controversial paper in the *Lancet*, showed that men from social class five whose wives had a very high rate of cervical disease, also had very high levels of sperm basic protein, especially protamine, and that men in social class one and two had low levels. The paper was accepted in the *Lancet*, raised obviously a lot of ethical problems, but he did show that there was a profound difference between the social classes on that subject.[79] These substances profoundly influence cell surface function *in vitro*. He then went ahead and in 1987 showed indeed in tissue culture work that you could imitate most of the morphological features of malignant cells. He did time-lapse photography and showed that adding protamine, which is a basic protein to the cell structures, when added to the cell cultures, induced these changes. During the 1970s, many of us still believed that DNA in some form, be it in viral form or in the actual virus or indeed sperm, was responsible, and I wrote a letter to the *BMJ* on the 11 October 1969, which is 39 years ago, to an article on contraceptives and cervical cancer, and said that these steroids could prevent the entry of the proposed genital mutagen, be it in the form of 'spermatozoal or viral DNA'.[80] Then Rawls and Melnick published their work on herpes simplex virus 2 (HSV-2) in Houston in 1968.[81] But again we pointed out that probably there was more DNA from sperm origin than there was from viral. So there was quite a lot of activity in that field on the male.

---

[79] The data from Reid *et al.* (1978a) were re-cast in Reid *et al.* (1978b) as a result of the suggestions from Cameron and Jones (1978): 366, and showed a higher degree of significance than reported in the earlier paper.

[80] Singer *et al.* (1969).

[81] Rawls *et al.* (1968).

I came to England and was influenced by the lady sitting on my left (Valerie Beral). We had both been residents in Australia at the same hospital many years before and she published a classic paper in 1974 on the standardized mortality ratio for cervical cancer by social class and husbands' occupation in married women.[82] If you were a fisherman, your wife would have had a standardized mortality ratio (SMR) of 257, or the wife of a driver of road goods vehicles of 168; compared to the Oxford clergyman's wife who was 12, or a scientist's wife who was 17 (Table 2, page 32). And on the basis of that and knowing what we knew about some of the basic work, Bevan Reid and Malcolm Coppleson joined me in writing a hypothesis published in the *American Journal of Obstetrics and Gynecology* on the role of the high-risk male in the aetiology of cervical cancer, a correlation of epidemiology and molecular biology.[83] Certainly Stanley Way gave me some of his anecdotal comments to add to that. The high-risk male as we suggested was determined by occupation, as Valerie had pointed out: sexual behaviour, cigarette smoking, sexually transmitted infection (STI), and genital HPV infection.

I came down to London from Sheffield in 1980 and met David Oriel at University College Hospital (UCH), who was a world expert on genital condyloma, and over the next few years he allowed a team comprised of Michael Campion and other research fellows to study the relationship between cervical and penile condyloma. Jack Cuzick and Dennis McCance also helped us and we published a number of papers showing that the women whose partners had penile HPV were at a very increased risk of cervical disease.[84] So that is really the unknown male factor. It started off being unknown, because the only work before the 1960s dated back to 1842 to Rigoni-Stern, who showed that nuns had a low rate of cervical cancer, and married and widowed women had a high rate of cervical cancer.[85] Very little occurred in the 1950s. Isadore Rotkin wrote on female behaviour, on the early age of first intercourse;[86] but it wasn't until the sperm work and the HSV work developed that we started looking at the male and then eventually at warts in the 1980s.[87]

---

[82] Beral (1974): data on page 1039, see Table 2, page 32; see also Wakefield *et al.* (1973); Anon. (1973).

[83] Singer *et al.* (1976).

[84] Campion *et al.* (1985); McCance *et al.* (1985).

[85] Rigoni-Stern (1842, 1988); Griffiths (1991); Scotto and Bailar (1969); see also note 236.

[86] Rotkin (1962, 1973).

[87] Singer and Stevenson (1972); Singer (1983); Walker *et al.* (1983a).

Social class	Husband's occupation	SMR
I	All occupations	**34**
	clergymen	12
	scientists	17
	civil engineers	60
II	All occupations	**64**
	teachers	30
	senior government officials	40
	publicans & innkeepers	120
	lodging house & hotelkeepers	150
III	All occupations	**100**
	clerks of works	40
	clerks	64
	crane & hoist operators	159
	drivers of road goods vehicles	168
IV	All occupations	**116**
	shopkeepers & assistants	71
	gardeners & groundsmen	98
	fishermen	257
	deck & engineroom ratings, barge & boatmen	263
V	All occupations	**181**
	office & window cleaners	95
	labourers	222

Table 2: Standardized mortality ratios (SMRs) for cervical cancer in married women, by social class and occupation of husband, England and Wales, 1959–63. Beral (1974): 1039.

McCluggage: Well, that was a very complete summary of the unknown male factor. Has anybody any comments about the unknown male factor?

Dr Anne Szarewski: I wanted to emphasize, perhaps, the role that Albert Singer played in this. I think that women in general should be very grateful that he highlighted the role of the male in cervical cancer, I think because there was so much stigma attached to it all being a 'female thing'.[88] It was really Albert's unit, which I joined in 1986, that was greatly responsible for the shift in emphasis to say that: 'Actually this is a joint problem, it's not the fault of the woman'. I think that a lot of the research that went on in our unit helped that shift a great deal.

Miller: I wanted to comment that the epidemiologists had identified a male factor. There was a case control study published in the UK, I think Buckley was the first author, which showed this and there were several studies of epidemiologists

[88] Singer *et al.* (1976).

which showed that husbands whose wives had died of cervical cancer, their second wife was at a greater risk.[89] So there was a fair amount coming in the epidemiology area. Rotkin and various others were pointing out the importance of the male. While I am talking, could I point out that it was Alex Meisels, the cytopathologist in Montreal, who identified some of the cytological changes that later were found to be due to HPV.

Professor Margaret Stanley: There was no doubt that there was a male factor. The epidemiology that had been done in the first part of the century and in the 1950s showed that.[90] There were some very amusing reports in the literature. One of my favourites was of a guy in the US whose wife had cervix cancer and whose other partners lived within a relatively short distance also had cervix cancer.[91] My boss, James Kirkland – the best gynaecological pathologist I have ever known, who had trained as a cytopathologist under Elizabeth Macgregor and went to Hans Hinselmann where he was trained as a colposcopist – had a very wicked sense of humour and said: 'He didn't even need a bike.' So the male factor was known and it's about the sociological and cultural attitudes of the time that you would always blame women.

I remember being on a radio programme in Australia, where we were talking and I was being asked questions about cervical cancer. I trotted out the usual risk factors – early age of sex, usually more partners – and one lady phoned up in absolute fury, and she said that she had been married since she was 16, she had never had another partner, she had had five children, but her husband was a merchant seaman. I rest my case.

Patrick Walker: Before we move on to the science and the next bit, it is worthwhile remembering what it was like and how much HSV had actually dominated the agenda through the 1970s. I started working with Albert Singer in 1981 and he sent me along to Dulcie Coleman to work in the lab there, and HSV was very much 'it'. It was intriguing at the time, I went to a meeting where Laura Aurelian and Irvine Kessler came over to speak, and Ralph Richart was there as well.[92] By the very tail end of the meeting, they were struggling to

---

[89] Buckley *et al.* (1981).

[90] Rotkin (1967).

[91] Professor Margaret Stanley wrote: 'It was in the *American Journal of Obstetrics and Gynecology*, but the precise reference is not in my records.' Note on draft transcript, 1 September 2009.

[92] Richart (1964) introduced the terminology of cervical intraepithelial neoplasia (CIN).

keep the hypothesis of HSV going, and the difficulty was that they couldn't find the DNA of the virus in the malignant tissue. They found the RNA and therefore they developed something, I think McDougall called it 'the hit and run hypothesis' (the virus got in, did the damage and then ran away again). As our colleague (Anthony Miller) mentioned, Meisels, Fortin and Roy's paper at the same time as Eva Savia and E Purola in Finland were identifying cytopathological changes that could be HPV.[93]

It always seemed strange to me as a young man entering the field at the time that now we see koilocytosis and dyskeratosis everywhere, what were people looking at in the 1970s during the HSV era that all of this so obviously became true later?

Stanley: Cytologists did recognize these funny cells, but we called them halo cells, we didn't know what they were. They weren't regarded, and Dulcie Coleman may wish to comment. But I want to reinforce what Patrick Walker said, HSV utterly dominated the agenda, and it was very much based – and Joan Macnab may want to comment here[94] – on the serology and the relationship between antibody levels to HSV-2, but the thing that really should have killed it was that nobody could transform human cells in tissue culture, or primary cells other than rodent cells with HSV DNA or any fragment of HSV, and one has to remember that the transformation assays that were used to support the idea of HSV involvement were all done on Syrian hamster or mouse fibroblasts. Anybody who works on those knows you only have to spit at these cells and they will obligingly transform for you. So, that was the basis of the science.[95]

Dr John Smith: About the koilocyte: those of you who know the Papanicolaou *Atlas of Exfoliative Cytology* from 1954, will know that it contains these marvellous coloured pen-and-ink drawings of abnormal cells. There is a most fantastic illustration of a koilocyte there, though its significance, of course, was not realized at the time.

---

[93] Purola and Savia (1977); Meisels *et al.* (1977); see also Nieminen *et al.* (1991).

[94] Dr Joan Macnab wrote: 'I would like to record that the molecular analyses of cervical tumours in Glasgow confirmed that HSV DNA could be retained. Furthermore, HSV was re-activable from rat transformed cells using genetic techniques of analyses (Park *et al.* (1980, 1983)).' Note on draft transcript, 2 September 2008.

[95] See, for example, Galloway *et al.* (1980); Stern and Stanley (eds) (1994).

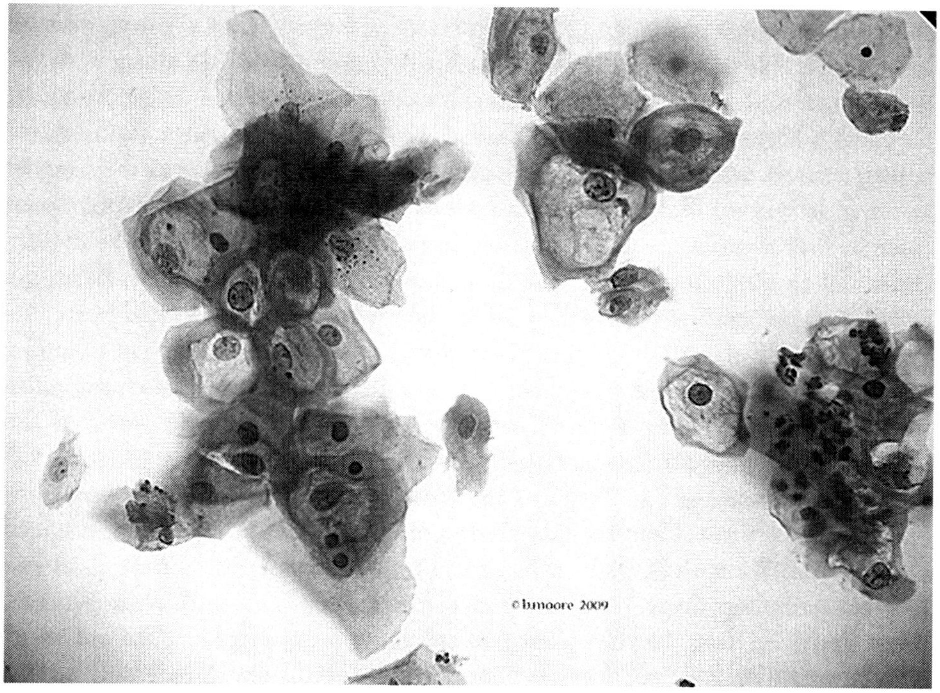

Figure 4: Koilocytes, cells infected with HPV
(400× magnification), stained with the Papanicolaou stain.[96]

McCluggage: That leads us on very nicely to the discovery of HPV16 and -18 as a major cause of cervical cancer and precancerous lesions, so again, Albert Singer.

Singer: I feel rather humbled talking on this topic that everyone here is so involved with. But again I start with Coppleson and Reid in 1966. It was obvious to us that age of first intercourse and of 'promiscuous adolescence' were very important as behavioural characteristics.

The first thing they got me to do was to start looking at the cervix of virginal girls and those of sexually active girls. Well, you will say, how can you look at virginal girls? In the 1960s it was usual for what was called the 'strip and stretch' of the hymen to be done under anaesthetic before a young woman married. And working in a big hospital in Sydney, Val Beral knows it well, many of

---

[96] 'Their form indicates a transition from the navicular to the superficial type. Cells exhibiting dyskaryotic changes...affect chiefly the nucleus and consist in enlargement, irregularity in form, hyperchromasia and bi- or multinucleation. In the superficial and navicular dyskaryotic cells a perinuclear "cavitation" is often present' (Papanicolaou (1954): A.VI.9, pages a14–a15).

the gynaecologists had huge private practices and every time a young woman came in for this procedure, I would ask for permission and run along with my colposcope, and in the space of about ten seconds was allowed to get a picture. So I had a library of the cervix of virginal women, and then the sexually active young women, and we published this and showed that the cervix of the sexually active girls was smaller, but that squamous metaplasia was very active, about three or four times more active, but the important thing was there was atypical abnormal epithelium present.[97] We then started to biopsy the cervix. Now, the population we studied was a group of women whom Coppleson had been able to observe, and these were young women in an institution who were offered a bacterial examination to exclude STI of the vagina, and during that examination we photographed. They were all sexually active, and I brought some of the original photographs taken at the time with me. We have Miss H, aged 14, sexual intercourse age 12. They had the most unusual changes in the cervix; we had never seen these. Coppleson couldn't work it out, and he was an experienced colposcopist. We took biopsies of these and I remembered photos from Koss and Durfee's pathology book.[98] So I sent him some of these black-and-white pictures. 'Dear Professor Koss, In your book you call these warty atypia. What are they?' And he wrote back – I still have the letter and Leo Koss has mine – and we had a correspondence. He said these are 'warty atypia'; this was 1968.

Then we had to work out these changes, and Coppleson said that indeed these were obviously very profound changes and held the key to the whole abnormal process in the cervix.[99] At the time the pathologists really didn't recognize it. I have a book from 1973 by Fred Langley and Archie Crompton on epithelial abnormalities.[100] There are four lines devoted to 'warty atypia', which were cells similar to these cells, which were obvious HPV.[101] Koilocytes were noted in the condyloma, thus suggesting a possible relationship to infection. However, Patten considered these

---

[97] Singer (1975).

[98] Koss (1961) was a 'Citation Classic' in *Current Contents: Life sciences* (1989) 32: 15, having been cited in over 1260 publications. See also Koss and Durfee (1956); Koss *et al.* (1963); Koss (1975).

[99] Coppleson (1970).

[100] The lines read: 'Cells similar to these are seen in condyloma acuminatum, thus suggesting a possible relation to virus infection. Indeed Koss (1968) terms these changes 'warty atypia'. However, Patten (1969) states that the perinuclear clear zone has been attributed to shrinkage and Sagiroglu (1963) considers it an artefact.' Langley and Crompton (1973): page opposite Fig.5.3a and b.

[101] Langley and Crompton (1973): Figure 5.2.

changes to be artefact and Langley himself said these were degenerative cells. But we believed that these changes all were related to viral infections.

An offshoot of the work was that we wanted to know how the virus, or what it was that was causing it, got into the cervix? Reid asked if the young woman ovulated soon after she starts having her periods? The answer was: 'No, young women don't ovulate for a few years after.' He said: 'Maybe there are structures in the mucus that allows the entry at that time.' Again we examined the structure on an electromicroscopy of cervical mucus and again the original picture showed, as you would expect, that at mid-cycle if you are not ovulating, you have very clear channels, and when you ovulate these channels are blocked. So, here was a possible mechanism by whatever it was 'got into'.

We then went on from that and really I wanted to see what happened to these girls as they got older. I came to this country and managed to link up with Sir Richard Doll, who directed two young research fellows, Martin Vessey and Peter Smith, to help me in a study at Holloway Prison (1970–73). I managed, and it's another whole story, to get into Holloway Prison, set up the colposcopy clinic and examine 768 women, 38 per cent of whom had CIN and for whom 18 per cent had CIN or cancer and the biopsy showed exactly the same result as we had previously.[102]

Jenkins: I think one of the key things, Albert, was when the probes began to arrive, with the setting up of Southern blotting techniques.[103]

Singer: If I may have ten seconds. Dulcie Coleman was helping me and we set up a study with Patrick Walker.[104] The main study that we did was in 1983 and Jack Cuzick was also involved. We wanted to know what happened to women with mild changes in smears, most of whom had an HPV infection. We followed these women for three years with no biopsy, and showed that 26 of the 100 with mild changes (CIN1) turned into severe disease (i.e. CIN2/3) and 85 per cent of these had HPV16. Dennis McCance at Guy's Hospital did the hybridization and, as far as HPV16 was concerned, that was really the turning point.[105]

---

[102] Subjects were from King George V Memorial Hospital, Sydney, Australia, and HM Prison, Holloway, London, with financial support from the National Health and Medical Research Councils in Australia and a project grant from the Medical Research Council, London (Singer (1975)). See also Singer (1973).

[103] Melchers *et al.* (1991); Tidy *et al.* (1989). See note 108.

[104] Walker *et al.* (1983a and b).

[105] Campion *et al.* (1986).

Professor Heather Cubie: I wondered if I could give a slight virologist's perspective and go back a little bit, too, because there was quite a lot of virology happening, looking at papillomaviruses in the 1960s, particularly in the Institute of Virology in Glasgow, and we were doing quite a bit in Edinburgh. Albert Singer has referred to what I actually think still is one of the sentinel differentiations, which was David Oriel and June Almeida's electron microscopy work, coupled with what Marie Ogilvie did in Edinburgh, to separate out genital wart virus from the virus causing cutaneous warts.[106] That was the first indication that perhaps there were different kinds of this virus, and through the second half of the 1960s, and the early 1970s, lots of work was done trying to find *in vitro* models, as Margaret Stanley has mentioned too, and cell culture systems which didn't work. I was much involved in those animal models, which were jolly hard to do.[107] Then molecular techniques came along, starting with things like hybridization with the most cumbersome of techniques, coupled with Southern blotting – again an Edinburgh discovery and yet hugely influential in being able to move forward to eventually produce knowledge about different types of HPV – and that was the late 1970s.[108]

I wonder if I could make one more interesting point? The first international papillomavirus meeting was in 1975 and was held in Lyons, organized by the Institute Pasteur dermatologists. And, there was the beginning of an association of papillomavirus with cervical disease in terms of the virology at that stage.[109]

Professor Saveria Campo: I wish to point out that the discovery of HPV16 and HPV18 was made in the laboratory of Harald zur Hausen in Heidelberg, and it was made possible because Lutz Gissmann cloned HPV6 from a genital condyloma and used that molecular clone of HPV6 as a probe.[110] They were the ones that found HPV16 and -18 in SiHa and CaSki cells, and then they found them in several biopsies of cervical cancer, so we mustn't forget that they actually found for the first time HPV viral DNA in cervical cell lines and in cervical cancer specimens.[111]

---

[106] Dunn and Ogilvie (1968); Oriel and Almeida (1970). See also note 84.

[107] Cubie (1976).

[108] Southern (1975).

[109] Prunieras (ed.) (1976).

[110] Gissmann and zur Hausen (1980); Dürst *et al.* (1983); Boshart *et al.* (1984).

[111] zur Hausen *et al.* (1974); Gissmann and zur Hausen (1976).

Stanley: I want to reinforce that and to also point out that zur Hausen had published a paper early in the 1970s, where he had been looking for papillomavirus DNA in cervical cancer biopsies.[112] And the problem was that the molecular technologies were not advanced enough at that point for him to do it, and it wasn't until 1978, when Gissmann cloned HPV11.[113] This was absolutely critical, because without that, then the actual cloning out of HPV16 and HPV18 would not have happened and that was crucial. Lionel, who knows more about this perhaps than anyone else in the room, might want to comment.

Dr Lionel Crawford: I think the main comment is that I wish that Lutz Gissmann was here because I think he could really fill us in on the logic of what they did and the technology behind it. Certainly zur Hausen's lab was extremely important in all of this and continued to be for a long period. So his is a name which should be very prominent in all of these studies. If I could make a perverse comment at the same time: zur Hausen's generosity in giving everybody clones so that they could do searches with his cloned material had an unfortunate effect. This turned out to be a standard that everyone was using and the standard had in it a mutation which was effectively an assembly minus lesion which made it more difficult to assemble L1 into virus particles. In a way people would have been better off to isolating their own strains and later on it was found in my lab and Gissmann's lab that most of the natural isolates differed from zur Hausen's clone in a position in L1 which is critical, because L1 is the major coat protein.[114]

McCluggage: Thank you for that. We are going to move on to Dr Campo, who is going to talk about the mechanisms and genes of HPV.

Campo: I work in Glasgow, and the reason I work there is because at the end of 1978 I read a review by Bill Jarrett, who was a veteran pathologist, on the fact that BPV, bovine papillomavirus, was the cause of upper gastrointestinal tract cancer.[115] And I thought, 'Hey, this is a real cancer virus'. I was working on SV40 and was absolutely fed up with working on SV40 because I couldn't see where this was going to lead me. I wrote Jarrett a letter saying: 'You have a

---

[112] zur Hausen *et al.* (1974).

[113] Dartmann *et al.* (1986).

[114] Dr Lionel Crawford wrote: 'I learned at this meeting that the sequence of the L1 gene in the patent application is not that of the zur Hausen HPV16 clone, so this point may be irrelevant to VLP production mentioned later.' Note on draft transcript, 16 July 2008.

[115] Jarrett *et al.* (1978a and b); Jarrett (1978).

system and I have the molecular techniques, so why don't I come and work with you?' And he said: 'Yes, sure, come on.' And the rest of it is history. I went to Glasgow and stayed there.

To go back to HPV. As I have said, HPV was discovered later. In fact BPV was one of the first cancer viruses, papillomavirus-induced cancer. It was found along with CRPV, the cotton-tail rabbit papillomavirus, and these were the days when, as has been said, nothing was known about HPV16 or HPV18.[116] It was really thought that these were different viruses from genital condyloma and all the studies were being done on the rabbit and the bovine virus. Anyway, talking about the mechanisms of HPV: if we take HPV16 as the paradigm, then this virus has three transforming proteins that contribute to cervical cancer formation and these are: E5, E6 and E7. It is now accepted that E6 and E7 are the major transforming proteins and E5 is an auxiliary transforming protein.[117] The thing that fascinates me is that there are viruses, a whole lot of HPV viruses, that do not have E6, like BPV4, and they are perfectly good at inducing tumours and inducing cancer. And there are viruses that do not have E5, so whatever E5 does – and we can talk about what E5 does later – these viruses can do without E5 altogether. There is a whole class of bovine viruses again, in which E7 does not bind the protein pRB, which is what HPV16 E7 does. So whereas all these proteins undoubtedly do their thing in the transformation of cervical keratinocytes, there are an awful lot of viruses that can do without one or the other of these proteins. So I find this is actually quite interesting and perhaps these viruses should be studied more. These proteins that operate on cell transformation by pushing the accelerators, disabling the brakes, preventing apoptosis, these very same proteins are those that disable the immune response. They interfere with the immunomolecules of the host and they practically make the infected cell, the HPV cell, invisible to the host lymphocytes. So, it's a very clever system for such a small virus, it encodes two or three proteins that can do multiple things: one is to put the cells into proliferation and at the same time prevent the host's immune system from recognizing cells that are proliferating when they shouldn't.

Dr Joan Macnab: I think that's interesting, but in my lab Henry Kitchener, John Murdoch and Steve Walkinshaw did a lot of work on cervical cancer with me. One of the issues we found – perhaps not common to the whole of the

---

[116] Shope (1933, 1937); Syverton (1952).

[117] Münger *et al.* (2004); Stöppler *et al.* (1996).

UK, but certainly to the west of Scotland – was the high incidence of HPV16 in normal samples. Initially HPV16 was found in cytologically normal tissue distant from a tumour, but later in CIN and in tissue from normal controls with no evidence of cytological abormality.[118] That made it very difficult for us as workers on HSV-2. We were in the position of having found HPV16 in a lot of circumstances that were difficult to explain. I think that HPV depends on other factors and has other aetiology in the patients in which it forms tumours. Co-factors could include HSV-2, which has proved to be present in cervical tumours, transformed cells and also to have the ability to increase expression of tumour-specific proteins such as the mitochondrial aspartate amino transaminase and up-regulate the oestrogen receptor.[119]

Crawford: May I speak up from the virus' point of view? There is no reason why the virus should care at all about transformation; it only cares about making more virus. It is perverse to only take the patient's point of view, whereas all the virus wants is to produce more and more virus. So the fact that it appears in normal cells, produces virus progeny, goes on to infect and everything else, that is fine. If occasionally there is transformation, it doesn't matter to the virus, but it matters a lot to the patient and to the doctor in charge. But I think one has to look at things from a different point of view to understand the way the virus works. So a lot of the things we have been talking about would not have interested the virus at all.

Jenkins: This issue of HPV in normal women is one of the things that has caused immense confusion, hasn't it? In terms of the development of the understanding and the impact of the papillomavirus, the finding of virus everywhere did for a while lead to considerable doubts about the oncogenic role of HPV and had a big impact on the whole research activity, research programmes, going on at that time in the 1980s.

Campo: I absolutely agree with every word that Lionel Crawford has said: the virus wants to make more of itself, and it doesn't care about cancer, which is a dead-end. Also, viruses are 'latent', can be latent, and papillomavirus has been found in normal margins of lesions; it has been found in epithelia away from lesions; it's been found in clinically normal people; and this is particularly problematic for skin cancer. I know that we are not talking about skin cancer

---

[118] Macnab *et al.* (1986); Kitchener *et al.* (1991).

[119] Lucasson *et al.* (1994); Offord *et al.* (1989).

at this meeting, but non-melanoma skin cancer is a point of controversy as far as HPV is concerned, precisely because the cutaneous squamous cell or basal carcinomas are also found so frequently in clinically normal skin. But that doesn't mean to say that once in a while an accident happens which is not good for the virus, it's not good for the host, but it's good for the transformed cell that gets selected then moves on.

Professor Julian Peto: I slightly disagree with Lionel. HPV16 is so extraordinary compared with other HPVs, in terms of its transformation power that something approaching half of all untreated women with HPV16 may develop CIN3. The consequence is that they remain infectious for much longer, so in the case of HPV16, you could argue that there has been selection for transformation, because it substantially increases the time that the carrier remains infectious in an unscreened, untreated population.

Jenkins: A lot of this has taken a long time to be understood, hasn't it? We are going back to the early days of looking at HPV. We were really unaware of a lot of these complications and the discovery of HPV in normal tissue as well as in cancerous and precancerous tissue did cause quite a stir and a lot of concern at the time, against the importance of HPV as an oncogenic agent.

Stanley: The problem with HPV was that infectious disease physicians and microbiologists were not much involved with it. It was gynaecologists and histopathologists, who really had very little understanding of infection and infectious disease, and that has always been a problem in the HPV field. The idea that with pathogens, with viruses, with any form of microbe, lots of people are exposed, lots of people are infected, relatively few actually show any clinical symptoms and really very few show the most severe and acute form of disease caused by the pathogen. That is as true of HPV as it is of even polio, for goodness sake.

Professor Ciaran Woodman: Somebody has to disagree with you, with the soundbite that 50 per cent of women with HPV16 develop CIN3; it's too large, much too large. We started on our own longitudinal studies which attempted to define a cohort in which we could measure the incidence of HPV16 and -18 infection, and the proportion of those who acquired the HPV16 infection soon after the onset of sexual intercourse was of an order of magnitude less than 50 per cent.[120]

---

[120] Tierney *et al.* (1993).

Crawford: *p53* is a whole meeting on its own, so I will only talk about it very briefly.[121] It has a very interesting history and came out of confusion, misunderstanding and SV40.[122]

But I will talk about virus-like particles (VLPs) and I find myself in the minority again, not speaking about the virus, but about prevention at a much earlier stage than detecting early lesions and removing them. My position, for the sake of argument, is that we could do without all of this if we had a decent vaccination system, and the basis of that has to be the virus coat protein and virus-like particles.[123] You see them in all sorts of wart virus, you see them in sections and in negative staining, they are particles which lack DNA, and, of course, you want anything that you are going to use to put into people to be devoid of DNA, because that removes all the worries about actually causing the disease, rather than preventing it. VLPs have been around for a long time, but producing them in quantity was felt by experts to be almost impossible. Even harmless sorts of warts, like the ones you get on your hands or your feet, couldn't be reproduced in the sort of quantity of virus required and then the empty particles separated out from the full particles, on a scale that would allow you to do anything useful. For the important viruses like HPV16 and -18, it was even more ridiculous, you couldn't get anywhere near it. There were certainly people who felt that the infection of epithelial cells in the state of terminal differentiation was essential for the production of virus particles, but this was not true.

The name I want to emphasize here is Jian Zhou (1957–99).[124] He felt that if you hooked up the virus coat protein gene (L1) to a strong enough promoter in vaccinia virus you could actually get it expressed in quantity in cells, not in terminal differentiation. He had survived the cultural revolution in China (1966–69)[125] and when he came over to the UK he was able to show that not only could he produce decent quantities of HPV16 L1 but he could also show that in mice there was a tissue-mediated immune response. When he went to

---

[121] For an overview, see Thomas *et al.* (1999).

[122] Levine (1976, 1990); Basilico (1984); Matlashewski (1989).

[123] See, for example, Zhou *et al.* (1990, 1992, 1994).

[124] Dr Jian Zhou discovered the HPV VLPs (Zhou *et al.* (1991)) that enabled the development of the cervical cancer vaccines *Gardasil* and *Cervarix*. See Figure 5, note 127 and Biographical note on page 144.

[125] See, for example, Unschuld (1985); Ebrey (1996).

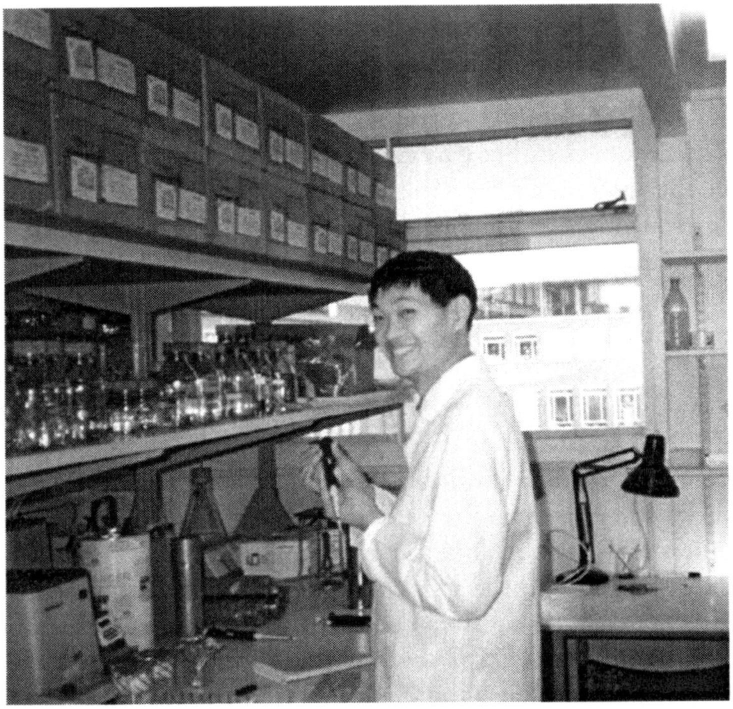

Figure 5: Dr Jian Zhou (1957–99) in Dr Lionel Crawford's laboratory, Cambridge, *c.* 1989.

Australia he continued this work and was able to produce VLPs. Admittedly they were sloppy for the reason that I have already mentioned, because we were generously given the HPV isolate from zur Hausen and that was the one being used. But I think this was very much where the whole vaccination story begins and I wish that Jian was here.

[Professor Valerie Beral asked about Zhou and Ian Frazer. She had thought VLPs were first produced by Ian Frazer].

Crawford: Jian had been out picking melons in the fields during the cultural revolution in China, and when he was allowed back into the lab he started to put together vaccinia constructs in which various proteins were expressed, in positions within the vaccinia genome where the promoter activity was extremely strong. One of those was L1 from HPV, and he wrote to me and asked if he could come to the lab. After a lot of coming and going – it was also the time of the general postal strike in 1971, which didn't make life any easier – he came over to my lab and continued this work. Jian and his wife, Xiao-yi Sun, were used to working extremely hard and doing everything for themselves, they worked like crazy and moved fast. So, to my mind, Jian was the person who was able to generate substantial amounts of L1, although not at this stage as virus-like. He also felt that the important thing was not to get humoral immunity, which you can get with bacterially produced L1, but also to put it into mice to get cytotoxic T cells, which he did.

Ian Frazer was in Margaret Stanley's lab next door during this time and we were having great difficulty in getting any sort of guarantee that we were going to get a passport for Jian since the Home Office wouldn't do anything. They said he could apply after several years' residence and that they would think about it. With the state of politics in China, he really needed a passport. Because the Australian authorities were much more flexible about this, he felt that he should get himself an Australian passport and be free to go wherever the good science was. When he got to Brisbane he continued that work and was able to produce pictures of VLPs, which sedimented in about the right region. They were clearly sloppy; they weren't really nice. Papillomaviruses are extremely pretty, they are beautiful things, but his were far from beautiful. They had all the main requirements, and as soon as you changed over the system, used a different sequence, without the assembly lesion, then you started getting good quantities of good particles. Other groups in the US also did similar things with papillomaviruses in all sorts of other systems.[126] I think the important breakthrough was the idea that if you put the L1 gene behind a really strong promoter, all the other requirements could be forgotten. And that turns it into a practical possibility. My feeling is – again I suppose I am disagreeing – that screening and everything else is all very well when you can afford it, but the vaccination of boys and girls worldwide seems to me to be the way to go in the long term, to get herd immunity at the stage of not being virus-infected, rather than becoming virus infected and then catching it at the eleventh hour or so.

> [Professor Valerie Beral asked Dr Lionel Crawford for clarification about who discovered VLPs, which was the breakthrough that led to the HPV vaccine.]

Crawford: Jian Zhou.

Cubie: I am so delighted that you have said all those things about Jian. He certainly was a very important person and I was privileged to be the person who was chairing a session, again at one of the international meetings, where

---

[126] University of Rochester, Georgetown University and the National Cancer Institute. See also note 127.

Jian presented his first revelation in 1991 in Seattle. Indeed, I have often been chased by the patent attorneys to give the exact timing of that presentation, and therefore from the historical point of view it was a very important thing to be associated with.[127]

Crawford: It was brilliant and that's why I have made such a point of it. Because, I think, one needs to acknowledge the people – in spite of all the difficulties and all the interference, political and otherwise – who knew what was important, and did it.

Stanley: Lionel is absolutely right. I have come back from Australia where we held the ninth anniversary of Jian's death (2008), and we really talked a lot about this.[128] I think Jian did something incredibly important and he drove it; he showed the particle and that there was activity. People had made VLPs for other viruses; in fact, the hepatitis B vaccine, which was developed and is being administered, is actually a VLP-like structure. So there were other people thinking about it and doing it. The baculovirus expression system for HPV was started in a PhD by Bob Rose in Rochester in the late 1980s,[129] but Jian was the first person to actually publish and show a VLP.[130] I think it needs to be recognized that the intellectual discussion and drive originated in Lionel's lab, and perhaps that hasn't been given the recognition it should.[131]

McCluggage: Can we move on to immune responses to HPV?

Stanley: Immune responses to HPV languished for a long time and it's important to say that pretty well everything we could understand about the immune response to papillomaviruses came from animal viruses. If you think about it, the first demonstration that a vaccine would work was done in 1937

---

[127] For the 2007 decision of the US Court of Appeals for federal circuit 2006-1154, interference no. 104,776, see www.cafc.uscourts.gov/opinions/06-1154.pdf (visited 6 October 2009). The work of Zhou *et al.* (1991) was not disputed. See also McNeil (2006).

[128] A memorial volume from that meeting is freely available at www.scribd.com/doc/2740521/zhou-jianprefaces-Etc (visited 23 April 2009).

[129] Rose *et al.* (1994a and b).

[130] Zhou *et al.* (1992).

[131] Dr Lionel Crawford FRS was made an honorary member of the Biochemical Society in 2004 and awarded the Royal Society's Gabor medal in 2005 for his work on the small DNA tumour viruses, specifically the papova virus group, papilloma, polyoma and SV40. For a description of his work, see www.biochemist.org/bio/02606/0063/026060063.pdf (visited 27 October 2009).

by Richard Shope, with the cotton-tail rabbit papillomavirus (CRPV).[132] The reason why Shope could do it was that you make a lot of virus in the cotton-tail rabbit, and so you could always extract the virus, which was pure, so you could challenge animals and show that the virus was infectious and would generate lesions. You could do the classic neutralization assays, which are the meat and drink of the virologist. In other words, have you generated an antibody response which will neutralize the virus and prevent it from infecting? You could do that in rabbits and cows. In 1937 Shope did a classic experiment. He took cotton-tail rabbit papillomavirus and he immunized the animal systemically. In other words, he infected intramuscularly. Not surprisingly, the animals didn't develop papillomaviruses, because you have to infect the skin if you are going to generate a papillomavirus lesion or wart. Even though the animals didn't make warts, they generated antibodies and Shope could show that this was neutralizing antibody in a classic method. What he then did was to take his immunized animals and tried to challenge them with virus. The immunized animals did not get warts, the non-immunized animals did. Now that is a classic experiment. It shows that if you can generate a neutralizing antibody, you will prevent infection with the virus.

You had to wait for the VLPs before the production of properly folded protein, because you have to have the protein folded to generate neutralizing antibodies. It took from 1937 to 1991 before the reagents were around to be able to test, if you like, the Shope experiment with HPV. The serology of HPV was useless until 1991, because we didn't have the proper reagents to measure circulating antibodies, so we couldn't do the standard things you would expect to do: looking at serum responses, antibody responses, to HPV. The other arm of the immune system, of course, cell-mediated immunity, was easier to attack, in the sense that we could make the proteins, we could make peptides and so we could start to ask questions about whether there were cytotoxic T-cell responses, whether it was a standard type of cell-mediated immune response to viruses, in other words mediated by CD8 T-cells. Here again, the virus was very difficult, because systemic responses to papillomaviruses turned out to be almost undetectable. Everybody struggled like mad in the 1980s, particularly to demonstrate that you could have a systemic response to HPV, either in terms of antibody, or in terms of T-cell. The antibody story took off as soon as we had VLPs, because you then had the right thing to measure. We are still struggling

[132] Shope (1937).

in 2008 with the cell-mediated response to HPV. We know it's important, we know the clearance of lesions is regulated by CD4 TH1-type responses, we still don't know what the primary cellular immune response to the virus-infected cell is. There are only two things you can say: that prophylactic vaccination works, because it has been demonstrated, but immunotherapy – which is the other thing that people want to generate – is very difficult because we don't understand how you clear the virus.

Campo: If I can take up this last point and continue with it. The strange thing is that therapy, therapeutic vaccination, works in the animal system: it works in the rabbit, it works in the cow, it works in the dog. There is something that we do not know about HPV in humans, which has prevented an effective therapeutic vaccination in humans. Every time we hear of a new trial: 'Yes, it works; it's very promising.' We have to continue. But still it is nothing like a preventive vaccine, the prophylactic vaccine which we are talking about that is 100 per cent effective. Any therapeutic vaccine against HPV is not as good as therapeutic vaccines against animal papillomaviruses, would you say? You [Margaret Stanley] have done therapy in the dog, we have done therapy in the cow and it works.[133]

Stanley: The trouble is that the therapeutic approach in humans is always targeted to precancerous lesions and therefore it becomes an anticancer vaccine rather than a therapeutic vaccine against a virus infection.

Cubie: There's another dimension to looking at immune responses, and that's clearly in epidemiological studies in large numbers. As we go towards the introduction of the vaccination and a lot of what we were talking about earlier, about the cytology and the colposcopy, I think it's really important to know how ubiquitous these papillomaviruses are, and, as Margaret said, once the VLPs were available we could do some extended serological work. Margaret and I worked on a group of children and found an incidence of antibodies to HPV16, not a very high incidence, about 7 per cent, compared with about 50 per cent of the kids having antibodies to the skin types.[134] Now, to me, that is a really important thing, because although the viruses that we are talking about in relation to cervical disease are being considered as sexually transmitted viruses, and the virus is undoubtedly usually sexually transmitted, it is possible to pick up that infection – whether it ever progresses to pathological disease –

---

[133] Campo *et al.* (1993); Moore *et al.* (2003).

[134] Cubie *et al.* (1998).

by nonsexual routes. It was serology as well as DNA detection that was able to show that.[135]

McCluggage: We are going to move on to Professor Peto, who is going to talk about the epidemiology, natural history and importance of HPV.

Peto: It was clear to everybody who was interested in HPV by about 1985 or 1986, that this was the cause of cervical cancer. It took us ten years to persuade the rest of the world, and a lot of clinicians were still sceptical until quite recently. It's extraordinary how suddenly things changed. Dulcie Coleman and I set up a cohort of 50 000 women in Manchester, and similar studies were done by many other people.[136] These large, population-based studies of women undergoing routine screening showed that about 20 per cent of women aged 20–24 had oncogenic HPV, not HPV6/HPV11, but the oncogenic types. It really was rather extraordinary. And it also became clear from such studies that most of these were transient infections, implying that something of the order of 50 per cent of the British female population were being infected with the virus that causes cervical cancer by the time they were 30. Everybody in this room knew this for 20 years, but it didn't become generally known until five years ago.[137] Those studies also showed the relationship between HPV and CIN3, although the relationship between HPV and cancer is more difficult to demonstrate in prospective studies because you have to wait so long and have so many people in the study. Ciaran Woodman described it as a soundbite, but in our cohort,[138] the cumulative risk of CIN3 in women with high-risk HPV and normal cytology was 28 per cent after 14 years.[139] That's why I questioned Lionel's comment that transformation is irrelevant to natural history, at least for HPV16. At that level I think it could appreciably affect viral evolution. Anyway, studies of that sort demonstrated the prevalence of HPV, but the fact that most infections disappear within two or

---

[135] Professor Heather Cubie wrote: 'Probably the most relevant work came from Drs Jenny Best and John Cason working at St Thomas' Hospital in studies on primary school children. Also work done in South Africa by Dr Dianne Marais, and by Dr Stina Syrjänen in Finland on family transmission studies, would also be useful.' Letter to Mrs Lois Reynolds, 9 September 2009. See Rice *et al.* (1999); Marais *et al.* (1997); Syrjänen and Puranen (2000).

[136] See also Wakefield *et al.* (1973).

[137] Zimet *et al.* (2006); Savard (2006).

[138] Peto *et al.* (2004b).

[139] Professor Julian Peto wrote: 'The CIN3 risk is much higher for HPV16 than for other high-risk types and the 28 per cent doesn't include CIN3 diagnosed at entry in cytologically abnormal women.' E-mail to Mrs Lois Reynolds, 5 November 2009.

three years is still slightly mysterious. Everybody has always had the idea that these were underlying chronic infections and nothing to worry about.

Something which has emerged quite recently is that the progression to high-grade disease appears to happen much more rapidly than was previously assumed. It may actually develop within two or three years, or not at all, as a consequence of recent infection. As we are only going up to 2000 in this Witness Seminar and this evidence has appeared in the last eight years, I think that the defects in cytology historically were really very considerable. The progressive improvement in cytology, particularly with re-training together with the introduction of LBC, has raised the sensitivity of cytology to about 95 per cent for detecting CIN3. It used to be less than 50 per cent in a lot of places. In the surveys that Jack Cuzick did in various centres around Europe, the sensitivities varied from about 30 per cent to 80 per cent not so long ago. Now it is over 90 per cent and there's very little difference between the sensitivity of HPV testing and cytology. CIN3s were often missed by screening, so you used to have to screen women again and again so that they were picked up eventually. Modern cytology is extraordinarily sensitive. We detected about 300 CIN3s at entry in 'A Randomized Trial In Screening To Improve Cytology' (ARTISTIC) trial, and we only detected ten extra CIN3s by testing everybody for HPV and colposcoping women still positive a year later.[140] So my view of the natural history of HPV has changed quite dramatically in the last five years. The improvements in cytology that have taken place quite recently have revealed a very different pattern from what we thought.

Professor Peter Sasieni: Rather than debating the natural history with you, here is an anecdote on the history. I was asked to give a talk at the Royal College of Obstetricians and Gynaecologists in the mid-to-late 1990s, I don't remember exactly when. I think it was David Luesley who was chairing it and decided at the end of it to say: 'Let's take a vote to see who believes that human papillomavirus is the cause of cervical cancer?' I lost the vote. It wasn't overwhelming, but I think about 60 per cent of the obstetricians and gynaecologists in the audience did not believe then that HPV was the cause of cervical cancer. It's interesting, because you were saying earlier, Albert, about koilocytes and HPV morphological changes, and I think that for that audience it was one of the reasons why they didn't believe that HPV was the cause. Because they were so used to seeing reports of HPV changes on smears, and knowing that it wasn't particularly relevant to high-grade disease, high-grade CIN, so although it was important,

---

[140] Sargent *et al.* (ARTISTIC study group) (2008).

the actual labelling of koilocytes as HPV changes could have had a detrimental effect, in terms of convincing most gynaecologists that HPV was the cause.

Jenkins: I think it is only since vaccination has begun to be studied clinically and to be promoted that the general public has really begun to accept, and I would include in that the vast majority of medical professionals, outside the small number of *cognoscenti*, that HPV is the causal agent of cervical cancer. Again, another personal statement: my daughter was taught in medical school, about five years ago, that HPV was thought by some people to be associated with cervical cancer, but nobody was sure about it. She came and questioned me on this, about what I had been doing for the last 20 years. These things did go on.

Singer: Patrick Walker failed to remember that we, along with Dennis McCance, wrote an editorial for the *BMJ*, 'Genital wart virus infection: nuisance or potentially lethal?'[141] That was more than 20 years ago, and, like you, I was ambushed at the Royal College of Obstetrics and Gynaecology in a 1988 debate entitled 'More people live off than die from HPV'.[142] That was less than 20 years ago, and 75 per cent of the audience believed that more people lived off HPV than died from it.

Peto: If you want to mention heroes in the history of HPV, Jan Walboomers, who unfortunately is also dead, was another extraordinary man. In the study which we initiated with the International Agency for Research on Cancer (IARC, part of the WHO), we collected cervical cancer specimens from nearly 1000 people in 22 different countries. They were looked at using the standard techniques for HPV detection and 93 per cent contained it. Jan re-analysed the negative samples and demonstrated that they all contained HPV. We finished up with only two out of 930 cancers that HPV was not isolated from. Jan's analysis was absolutely decisive in showing that HPV is present in essentially 100 per cent of cancers.[143]

McCluggage: The next session is about the UK national screening programme. I know there are several people from overseas and we would be very glad if they were able to comment on screening in other countries, but first Tony Miller will talk about evidence as to when screening works and when it does not.

---

[141] Singer *et al.* (1984); see also Singer and McCance (1985).

[142] Kitchener (1988).

[143] Walboomers *et al.* (1999).

Miller: Screening works when you get a high proportion of the at-risk population involved in screening. That, indeed, had been one of the big issues in this country (from our perception outside of the country). We were looking at this, as Jocelyn said earlier, in relation to the fact that Finland had initiated a programme in women aged 30 to 54 and achieved very high compliance, a most successful programme. Five-yearly screening had as much impact as in the US and Canada, where we had largely annual screening – and the reduction in mortality has been the same, 80 per cent in the US and Canada, 80 per cent in Finland, contrasting also with other Scandinavian countries, and with Norway particularly.[144] I think what became clear from outside as well as from what was done here, is that if you made a big impact on the population and invited the right sort of people to come in – and in fact I believe that the genius in this country was to use the NHS register for that purpose – it called in the women and you had the impact. I don't know how many people have looked at the international contrasts, but the contrasts between Finland, Canada, the US and the UK is the separation that occurred in the reduction, and the area between the curves, when the UK finally got its act together and the mortality came down. So you had this great gap between these countries, when mortality had not fallen in the UK, and when essentially a lot of women died as a result of not bringing forward screening.

I would like to come back to this issue of cytology sensitivity. It may well be true that there were some laboratories in the US, and maybe in the UK, which had 30 per cent sensitivity. In British Columbia, where we made some very good estimates, it was 75 per cent. Now 75 per cent is not what Julian said, he was talking about 95 per cent. But 75 per cent in the context of the amount of screening that was done clearly resulted in detecting the majority of the disease, which is progressive. The only other point I think I need to make is about when screening did not work, that there is still in every country this great divide between those whom we are able to bring to screening, and those we are not. The fact that we have a plateau in nearly all countries in terms of reduction of mortality, particularly in North America, has been because we haven't been able to bring recent migrants and people in the lower social classes into the programme. That's a lesson that I think has got to be borne in mind in terms of vaccination. When you hear in reports, as we have recently, that you only get 70 per cent compliance, that is 70 per cent of the 70 per cent effectiveness, and you are then below 50 per cent. So, I think we have to be extremely cautious when we look at this.

---

144 Hakama (1982); see also note 39.

I know we are not meant to go beyond 2000, but I want to make the point that we all have to bear in mind – and we are thinking about this very hard at the moment in Canada – that we have to set out our programmes for the future, ensuring that the vaccinated women get screened appropriately, and ensuring that the unvaccinated women still continue to get screened. So screening works when the women at risk are screened. And that is what you have got to do to ensure a successful programme.

Duncan: The Walton Report came out in 1976, and, of course, it was slightly counter-productive, because the women could select themselves whether they were high-risk or low-risk and be screened with a frequency which was different for the two categories.[145] There was a slight blip because all screening went down, because nobody wanted to point a finger at themselves, and say: 'I am "high-risk".' We have had difficulties in Scotland recently with younger women who are not coming for screening. It's a bit like HIV and all the protection for that. It's almost like wanton risk-taking when it is not due to ignorance. So, younger women are not coming for screening.[146]

We did look at a rural population and an urban population several years ago, trying to identify why women were not being screened. These were women who were approached up to eight times to find out why they were not coming. Many of them had been informed, or were well informed, and decided that they themselves were not at any significant risk. And so it's quite interesting how people absent themselves from the screening programme.

Sasieni: Of course, if you don't screen a woman, you are not going to do any good in terms of preventing cancer, but it's not enough to do a screening test.[147] As has been seen all over the world, it has to be an integrated programme. You have got to make sure that the women get the results of the smear, which doesn't happen in many cases. You have got to make sure that treatment is available, which doesn't always happen. In parts of Latin America, something like 80 per cent of women had a smear in the last three years. But if they have an abnormal smear, there is no treatment facility for them. They would have to fly to a major city to get treatment, which they can't do, so it's a total waste of time doing the smear tests. The quality of the smears is really poor, particularly because there are high rates of infection. So when you are looking on a global scale, there

---

[145] See note 48.

[146] Cockcroft (2009).

[147] Sasieni *et al.* (1996).

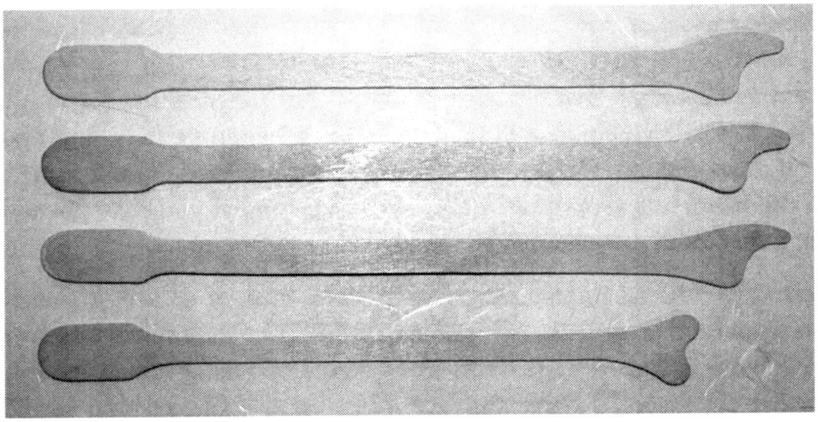

Figure 6: Three Aylesbury spatulas and one Ayre spatula, 2009.
The Ayre was the Department of Health spatula, replaced as the spatula of choice by the Aylesbury from 1984 onwards.

are a lot of reasons, a lot of factors, which are critical to making a screening programme work.

As Margaret Wolfendale is here we should think about the smear-taking device.[148] The extended tip spatula made a big difference in terms of the quality of the smears, and what you could detect: the Aylesbury spatula and a good laboratory.

I think that there are a lot of other factors. Of course, when you are not covering the whole population you cannot have a big impact. That was the big difference between Norway and Finland because, I think, they were taking a similar number of smears, but in Norway it was the same women who were being screened every year and in Finland they were making sure that they had very high coverage with five-yearly screening. So that is important. There is so much more to cervical screening than doing a smear test.

Herbert: I quite agree with what Peter Sasieni said. If there isn't good quality in all parts of the programme, it won't be effective. May I say two things: the first about Finland. Screening every five years from age 30–55 was always attractive to people organizing programmes elsewhere, but in Finland they do not register opportunistic smears – more than 50 per cent of smears were taken outside the organized programme.[149] So a lot of women would have been screened in

[148] Wolfendale *et al.* (1987); see in particular page 33 and Figure 6 above.

[149] Hakama (1990).

their twenties and might have had CIN3 treated. You can't assume from the programme in Finland that screening every five years between the ages of 30–55 is enough, because that was not what happened in practice.

The other point I want to make is that people may think that screening has had no effect when the risk of disease had changed.[150] All through the 1970s and 1980s, there were around 4000 cancers and 2000 deaths in England and Wales, and people said that screening hadn't made any difference at all. But if you look at CIN3 rates, there were increasing numbers of women being successfully treated and those women were at lower risk of getting cancer later in life. Because there was a younger birth cohort at greater risk and an older one in whom screening was to some extent working, it looked as though there was no effect. That is still happening in some places in Eastern Europe. Recently I showed the English figures for cancer incidence with the Czech figures superimposed over them and they are very similar to ours in 1985, when incidence was increasing.[151] Screening may appear not to be working because the cancer rates are unchanged, but its effect depends on whether the risk of disease was changing.

Chamberlain: I wanted to take up something that Peter Sasieni said about the lack of adequate treatment. I am quite surprised at this historical meeting that nobody has mentioned the New Zealand experience, where there was a gynaecologist called Herbert Green, who believed that screening was unnecessary because he maintained that precancerous changes did not progress, and so he set out to prove it by not treating women with what was then called cervical carcinoma *in situ*.[152] I actually met him once when I was working as a very junior assistant to Max Wilson, whom some of you will remember as one of the Department of Health people who argued early on for screening – Wilson of Wilson and Jungner's 'ten principles of screening', this spelled out the criteria needed for screening to be successful and was published way back in the early 1960s or maybe late 1950s. Anyway, Herbert Green came to see Max Wilson to tell him about his plans, and Max said: 'That's fine, so long as you do it as a randomized controlled trial comparing your untreated group with a treated group as the controls, with stopping rules and a data monitoring committee, so that everything is above board.' Had this actually happened, we would have

---

[150] Draper and Cook (1983).

[151] Data from Rob (2007). See also cancer registration statistics at: www.statistics.gov.uk/StatBase/Product.asp?vlnk=7720 (visited 23 July 2009).

[152] Cartwright (1988); Jones (2009).

known the natural history of carcinoma *in situ* and of all CIN much, much sooner and more clearly than we do even today. Unfortunately Green didn't have a control group, and lots of women in New Zealand went on to develop cervical cancer unnecessarily because of this.[153]

Peto: David Skegg in New Zealand has updated the follow-up on that cohort, and it is about to be published.[154]

> [Professor Valerie Beral said a major paper on the natural history of cervical neoplasia was published in *Lancet Oncology* in April.]

Peto: Forty per cent of untreated women with CIN3 develop cancer. So it is going to be shown at last.

Miller: I agree absolutely with what Peter Sasieni said; I should have said it myself. I want to come back though to the Finnish experience. The Finns have done quite a lot of good, looking at the impact of opportunistic screening versus their organized programme and there's no question that the opportunistic screening is *not* very important, because it's largely given to women who are outside the age range you want to get at. Let's face it, there's absolutely no point in starting screening at the age of 18, 19, 20. And they published this.[155] So, it is the organized programme which has had the impact, rather than the opportunistic screening. In terms of how far you can get away with five-yearly versus three-yearly or more frequent screening, I think the natural history we gathered from British Columbia was useful; Nick Day essentially looked at this and gave an answer to that many years ago.[156] There's no question that three-yearly screening was optimal and five-yearly screening still highly effective. I hope we don't go away with another impression, and some recent models done by Sue Goldie essentially confirm that.[157]

---

[153] For discussion of ten US surveys, see Wilson (1961); Wilson and Jungner (1968). For the ten principles of screening, see Glossary, pages 151–2.

[154] McCredie *et al.* (2008).

[155] Anttila *et al.* (2004); Barnabas *et al.* (2006). England withdrew cervical screening to the age range 20–24 in 2004, as a result of Sasieni *et al.* (2003), although screening of this age range continues in Scotland and Wales. See also Law *et al.* (1999); McGahan *et al.* (2001). Professor Anthony Miller wrote: 'There is not a direct Finnish assessment of age of start, it is just that they started at age 35 and this was as effective as programs in North America starting at 18–20.' E-mail to Mrs Lois Reynolds, 5 September 2009.

[156] See IARC Working Group on evaluation of cervical cancer screening programmes (1986).

[157] Stout *et al.* (2008); Garnett *et al.* (2006); Goldie *et al.* (2001, 2004).

Wolfendale: May I come back to what Amanda Herbert was saying about the risk? If you want to stop the growth of cervical cancer and if there is a higher risk of cervical cancer in the younger age group, then if the risk of cervical cancer in younger women is increasing, it is then very difficult in the early years of screening to reduce the overall incidence of cervical cancer. In the 1970s Martin Usherwood and I saw a very large increase in CIN3 in our patients in Aylesbury, in a population we had studied and screened since the early 1960s. We showed a tremendous increase in CIN3 very clearly and we felt that, although we were having great trouble in actually reducing the cervical cancer rate, we were in fact holding back what could essentially have been an epidemic.[158]

Cuzick: Coming back on the question of when screening works: I think it emphasizes the need for continual monitoring of the screening programmes and not process monitoring of the detection of cytological abnormalities, but, like any large-scale process, monitor it by actually looking at the failures. That means going back and carefully looking at every case who gets cervix cancer and determining why the programme failed. Was it lack of coverage? Was it an abnormality that was not picked up? Or was there a normal screening and the test did not detect any abnormality? Any programme that's going to be successful has to maintain this long-term monitoring function.

Herbert: We are doing a great deal of monitoring now. We should face the fact that peak incidence of invasive cancer is now in women aged between 35–39; 2005 was the first year when it was higher than in women over 60. In my experience, something like 70 per cent of those cancers in women in their twenties and thirties are screen-detected early cancers, which is an additional benefit of screening. I quite agree with Peter Sasieni that most of these young women have already been screened. Most of them are interval cancers.[159] There are fewer opportunities for preventing a cancer that develops at age 35 than at age 50, and a single smear may not detect every abnormality. If you go back over the history of the women with cancer who have previously been screened, there are quite a number with evidence of CIN3 fairly recently. It might have been

---

[158] Wolfendale *et al.* (1983); Peto *et al.* (2004a) calculated that cervical screening costs about £150 million per year in England and would prevent about 4500 deaths per year. The overall cost was thus about £36 000 per life saved and £18 000 per cancer prevented, comparing all screening against none.

[159] Dr Amanda Herbert wrote: 'Sasieni *et al.* (2003) and Herbert *et al.* (2009) both show that cancers in young women are often "interval cancers". Herbert *et al.* (2009) also show a strong association between interval cancers, younger age groups and early stage screen-detected cancers.' Note on draft transcript, 1 September 2009.

missed on a smear – while others had inadequate smears, or had failed to have their latest smear or had one six years rather than three years before. Some did not attend for a biopsy, or had treatment and didn't come back for follow-up. It tends to be CIN3 rather than CIN2 that was missed or not treated, often within the previous three or four years' diagnosis. So I don't think in a community like ours, when we have got to a stage when we are detecting early cancer and saving these young women's lives, we can possibly not screen them in the preceding decade of life without increasing the rate of more advanced cancer.[160]

[Professor Valerie Beral commented that cervical screening in the UK today is working very well.]

Sasieni: I agree that the UK screening programme is extremely effective, working very well, but to say that it is preventing 90 per cent of cervical cancer in the UK is not really realistic, if coverage is only 80 per cent. If you look at the proportion of women aged 25 to 64 screened at least once within the last ten or 15 years it goes up to over 90 per cent, but that's only for those aged 25 to 64 years. There isn't huge evidence that it is preventing cancer in the over-70s. I think, realistically, cervical cancer incidence would be two and a half times higher than it is, and mortality would probably be three or four times higher, but not ten times higher. It is very, very effective.

Herbert: If you look at the incidence in one of those first high-risk cohorts, born, say, in 1950, the ones who had increasing cancer rates during the 1980s, incidence was more than 30 per 100 000 at age 35–39. Their incidence had gone down 15 years later by about 70 per cent, to something like 10 per 100 000, when it would be expected to have increased towards a plateau, as Julian was saying. Peter has published a graph of mortality in different birth cohorts showing much the same thing.[161] Treating CIN3 and early cancer prevents invasive or more advanced cancer later in life. Women in their fifties and sixties now, who were screened when they were younger, have got a very low risk of disease.

McCluggage: We are now going to talk about the organization of a national programme and the screening centre.

Herbert: May I go back to when it started? As we have already heard, it was extremely haphazard in the 1960s, with arguments about whether it was going to work or not, and some of the people who were promoting screening probably

---

160 Sigurdsson and Sigvaldason (2007).

161 Sasieni and Adams (1999).

thought it was going to be more effective than it was. I think that's undoubtedly true, because the enthusiasts exaggerate the benefits and there was a certain amount of acrimony about anybody who suggested that it wouldn't work. That was said to be Cochrane's experience, when he suggested that it might not be so successful and people thought he was saying something terrible.[162] Of course, we all know now that it's not quite as effective as it might be if every case of CIN3 was immediately detected and effectively treated and are well aware of the problems and disadvantages of screening. While in England enthusiasts were trying to get it going and the Department of Health was distributing circulars without enough money attached to them, in Aberdeen, Macgregor and Baird got on with setting up their own programme.[163] In their 1963 article they made the comment that it was past the stage of needing a controlled trial. They went out with balloons for the children and took smears from the women. As has already been said, they achieved good population coverage, monitored the outcome (using punch cards rather than computers), published a case-control study in 1985 and provided evidence in the UK that screening worked.[164]

Meanwhile, back in England, where the government was reluctant to pay, some highly effective screening was being carried out. CIN3 rates show how much the likes of Liz Mackenzie, Erica Wachtel and Dulcie Coleman were achieving, although many of the smears were taken opportunistically from young women. We shouldn't only look at mortality and incidence rates, we should also look at CIN3 rates, which were available from 1971 and went up at a much higher rate than the additional number of women screened.[165] Margaret Wolfendale showed an increase in severe dyskaryosis on smears in young women,[166] which was similar to the increases that were being reported in CIN3 as well as invasive cancer incidence and mortality, which gave us among the highest mortality

---

[162] Professor Archie Cochrane wrote: 'I remember giving a lecture in Cardiff on screening in 1967 into which I introduced the (as I thought) innocuous phrase "I know of no hard evidence, at present, that cervical smears are effective". To my surprise I was pilloried in the local Welsh press, who quoted many anonymous colleagues who thought me a "dangerous heretic" and I received many abusive letters, some from colleagues.' Cochrane (1972): 26–7; see also Bryder (2008); note 44. For a review of screening procedures, see Cochrane and Holland (1971); Wilson *et al.* (1971); Macgregor and Teper (1974).

[163] Macgregor and Baird (1963).

[164] Macgregor *et al.* (1985).

[165] Herbert (2000).

[166] Wolfendale *et al.* (1983).

anywhere in the world in women under 35.[167] All that happened in the 1980s when it seemed as though screening wasn't working at all; hence Knox's article in the *Lancet*.[168] It was terribly badly organized and quality control was poor. I remember doing a small study in 1988 when I had always been told that 90 per cent of women with cancer had never been screened (it was a sort of old cytologist's tale). I looked at our cases and saw that, yes, that was true if they were over 50, but if they were under 50, about half of them had been screened. When we looked back at the smears, there were all these small dyskaryotic cells, glandular abnormalities and things that were not being picked up.[169] We massively improved our quality control, which Muir Gray facilitated before the screening programme began.[170]

I think much of the success of screening since 1988 was due to quality control. Of course, there was the introduction of a computerized national register, so that all women aged 20–64 could be invited every five years, including those who had never been screened. With the old system there was no way of 'calling' women, it was only 'recall', so you never got the ones who didn't turn up in the first place. But particularly we started re-screening negative smears, improved training of cytologists, BMS and pathologists and, for the first time, had standards for comparing practice between laboratories,[171] as well as guidelines for 'fail-safe' follow-up of women with abnormalities.[172] The colposcopists and cytologists got together and discussed discrepancies and, in Southampton where I was working, the critical thing for us was to look back at the smears of the women who had got cancer and CIN3 and that's when we saw what had been missed.

---

167 Peto *et al.* (2004a): 252.

168 Anon. (1985); see also Knox (1966).

169 Herbert *et al.* (2009).

170 Dr Elizabeth Mackenzie wrote: 'These local programmes were properly coordinated finally by the Department of Health, first by the charismatic Dr Muir Gray prior to becoming part of Julietta Patnick's breast and cervical screening empire. It is now, in my humble opinion, the most successful national screening programme. My choice of specialty was enjoyable and fulfilling and was ideally suited to a peripatetic existence. My only regret, however, was that it was a struggle to get our specialty recognized in the early days and, as a consequence, promotion to a consultant post was often pitifully slow.' Note on draft transcript, 26 November 2008. See Gray (1990).

171 Chaired by Dr Amanda Herbert and together with Dr Jane Johnson and Mrs Julietta Patnick, led a Royal College of Pathologists, BSCC, NHSCSP working party (RCPath *et al.* (1995), also known an ABC).

172 Pike and Chamberlain (1992).

There is a well-known graph in a *BMJ* article by Quinn *et al.* showing that suddenly in 1988, the coverage went up and the incidence went down,[173] but we know from Macgregor's work in Aberdeen that it takes seven years for incidence to go down.[174] It didn't magically go down because the screening programme was launched. It was because of all the things that happened during the 1980s: the gradual increase in coverage and quality control, so that incidence eventually started going down. It went down in all the age groups eligible for screening, in what Bray called a 'period-specific change', seen in countries such as the UK when organized screening started, which was enough to cope with the cohort-specific change.[175] In the US and Canada they didn't see an increase in cancer; it was only in places like Norway, New Zealand and England that there was an increase in invasive cancer in the 1980s. In Canada and the US, Finland and Scandinavia, there may have been an increase in CIN3, but not in cancer, because they were controlling it. So, I think that Julietta Patnick's group and Muir Gray need credit, particularly for quality control, and for improving communication, so that colposcopists, histopathologists, everybody got together and discussed the problems.[176] I think that cancer audit, as Jack has said, is probably one of the most important things to show us where things have gone wrong.[177] I think that with what is happening now, we probably have one of the best screening programmes in the world.

McCluggage: Do you think anything useful will come out of the National Cervical Cancer Audit, which is now up and running?[178]

Herbert: I am working on our own cases at Guy's and St Thomas' at the moment. We are seeing two things in particular: first, that most of the cancers in young women are screen-detected and not all of those are microinvasive, and second – an interesting finding that was the same as in Southampton – that it's the early screen-detected cancers that are more likely to be interval cancers. The

---

[173] Quinn *et al.* (1999).

[174] Macgregor *et al.* (1994).

[175] Bray *et al.* (2005a).

[176] See Patnick (ed.) (2008b).

[177] Dr Amanda Herbert wrote: 'Robertson and Woodend (1993) were among the first to look back at smears from women who developed cancer and pointed out that what has more recently been introduced as "rapid review" of negative and inadequate smears might allow many of these abnormalities to be noticed by a second screener.' Note on draft transcript, 1 September 2009.

[178] The National Cervical Cancer Audit was introduced in 2007. See Patnick (ed.) (2006).

audit is showing, as Valerie Beral says, that we are down to rock bottom.[179] We are down to the ones which you can't prevent, but may detect.

Chamberlain: I agree with what Amanda said about the importance of quality control and its contribution to the success of our present programme.[180] But, even more important than laboratory-based quality control monitoring – and I don't think Amanda gave quite enough emphasis to this – is the fact that all women in the whole country, or at least those registered with a GP, are now routinely invited for screening. It is this that achieves the high level of population coverage, which is vital.

The template for using the NHS Central Register for cancer screening was, in fact, developed in the context of breast, not cervical cancer, as the method used in the UK Trial of Early Detection of Breast Cancer starting in 1978.[181] And subsequently in the Forrest Committee report on implementing national breast screening, which came out in 1986, a year before the Intercollegiate Cervical Screening Report,[182] we recommended that this system be introduced nationally. In comparing the introduction of national screening for breast and cervical cancer in the late 1980s, Muir Gray made an amusing but very pertinent analogy, in which health authorities were likened to a person being told to knit a garment. In the case of breast cancer screening, they were given a clear knitting pattern, a new ball of wool and some needles, and even some money to pay the knitters, so all they had to do was get on with it. Whereas with cervical cancer screening they were presented with a worn-out 20-year-old cardigan full of holes and they first of all had to unravel the whole thing, then roll up the wool, find the needles and start knitting, all without any extra

---

179 Dr Amanda Herbert wrote: 'Incidence of invasive cancer now (2005–06: figures from www.statistics.gov.uk/StatBase/Product.asp?vlnk=7720 (visited 1 September 2009)) "peaks" in women aged 30–34 years, incidence in older women having declined steadily in all age groups screened. According to our experience in London (unpublished) and Southampton (Herbert *et al.* (2009)), cancers in these young women tend to be early-stage screen-detected interval cancers in women little older than the 20-fold higher peak (aged 25–29 years) of incidence of CIN3, which is recorded on the same statistics website.' Note on draft transcript, 1 September 2009.

180 Professor Jocelyn Chamberlain wrote: 'Indeed, Catherine Pike and I wrote one of the guidelines on this put out by the NHS Cervical Screening Programme in 1991.' Note on draft transcript, 31 July 2008. See Pike and Chamberlain (1992).

181 See, for example, UK Trial of Early Detection of Breast Cancer Group (1981).

182 Department of Health and Social Security (1986b); NHS Breast Screening Programme (1991). See also Sutton (1997).

resources.[183] It is to the great credit of all the disciplines involved that it is now so successful.

Cuzick: A brief comment: I think a crucial issue was this transformation from a policy to a programme before this reorganization. Screening was a policy and not a programme. In our 1984 paper we outlined the requirements for a programme, including that somebody needs to be in charge of a fail-safe system and monitor overall performance.[184] This, I think, did actually outline in print the issues that many other people had enunciated in the early 1970s and laid down the important requirements for a programme, which I think did have an effect on this restructuring.

> [Professor Valerie Beral said that there was evidence that screening did work. The CMO, Donald Acheson, had suggested putting the case for the prediction of cervical cancer incidence and mortality in England and Wales.][185]

Sasieni: Historically, Julietta Patnick did not become involved in the start of this programme. For a number of years it was Elaine Farmery, who chaired the National Coordinating Committee with Muir Gray.[186] It's very difficult to know what was most important in improving coverage, but at the time, in the early 1990s, I believed, and I still believe, that the GP payments were extremely important. They had a payments system whereby there were much greater payments per smear in the practice that had at least 50 per cent coverage and greater still with over 80 per cent coverage.[187] And, cynically, it's amazing how very few people got much higher than 80 per cent, but virtually everywhere – well, lots and lots of places – 80 per cent was achieved, and it had a knock-on

---

[183] 'Developing a breast screening programme was like knitting a cardigan at terrific speed. Developing a cervical screening programme will be like unravelling a cardigan, writing the pattern, knitting it again at terrific speed, while still wearing it.' Dr Muir Gray talking about the late 1980s in NHS CSP (2003): 5.

[184] ICRF Coordinating Committee on Cervical Screening (1984).

[185] Beral and Booth (1986).

[186] ICRF Coordinating Committee on Cervical Screening (1984); Sasieni *et al.* (1996).

[187] GPs are paid to encourage patients to participate in the cervical screening programme. The basic-payment target, under the GP contract of 1990, was 50 per cent or more of eligible patients screened in the previous five-and-one-half years and a higher payment if 80 per cent or more were screened (Department of Health (1989)). Between April 1990 and October 1993 the percentage of general practitioners reaching the 80 per cent target rose from 53 per cent to 83 per cent, while the percentage achieving neither target decreased over the same period from 15 per cent to 3 per cent. Austoker (1994).

effect of actually removing people who didn't exist from GP lists, because they realized that they could get paid more from reaching these screening targets, than from having dead people on their lists. So I think the GP payment was actually critical.

Coleman: I would like to dwell on that and say: 'Yes, it did'; and one can be cynical about GPs responding to this system of payment, but on the other hand, there was tremendous cooperation from the people on the ground who were actually involved in the cytology service. The pathologists and the screeners were willing to subject themselves to testing twice a year and they still do this today. They have assessors who come round and test one's competence to screen, right from the consultant down to the lowest level of cytoscreener.[188] You have to pass that test before you are allowed to screen. But I think that cooperation is quite extraordinary, because I don't think it occurs in any other specialist field.

Herbert: The cancer audit shows that it isn't all about reviewing the smears. I agree with Jocelyn Chamberlain that you have to look at the quality of the call-and-recall and also at what the GPs are saying to the patients, and not focus only on the lab.

Sasieni: We have heard quite a lot about this. The public health impact was perhaps first seen from the Finnish data. What was happening in the UK in the 1980s was that although cervical cancer mortality (the standardized mortality rate in this country) was falling by about 1.5 per cent per year and had been since the late 1950s, cervical cancer incidence was fairly static overall and was increasing rapidly in young women. That was mostly due to this epidemic of HPV infections with a knock-on effect on cervical cancer, which we have heard about, and it made it very difficult to determine what effect cervical screening that was being done outside of any organized programme was having. However you interpret that, there was a dramatic change: if you look at the trends around 1988 to 1990, the mortality within a few years was falling by something like between 4–6 per cent a year and it continued to fall at that sort of rate, really accelerating the decline. For the first time we were seeing a fall in the incidence and there was this phenomenon, which people have alluded to – which we called the 'hockey stick'. If one followed a cohort

[188] See, for example, 'Evaluation of Clinical Events (ECE): Guidance for assessors and trainees in histopathology' from the Royal College of Pathologists (2008), freely available online at www.rcpath.org/resources/pdf/histopathology_ece_guidance.pdf (visited 5 August 2009).

of women, one had seen incidence increase with age at least until aged 50. After 1990, instead of their incidences increasing with age, in every single cohort, as the women aged, their cervical cancer rates came down. So some dramatic effects could be seen.

The initial emphasis with the reorganization of the programme had been to monitor the process, which made sense because you can look at process measures very soon after starting a programme. In about 1989 or 1990, Jack Cuzick, Jocelyn Chamberlain and Muir Gray decided that we needed to look at the effectiveness of screening and we introduced these audits, to see where screening was failing.[189] In other words, why were women getting cancer despite the fact that there was this screening programme. We did not want to attribute blame but to try to understand why these things were happening: how many deaths were inevitable? How many might be prevented by modifications? As people began to see what was going on, and why some of the cancers were occurring, greater emphasis was on quality assurance throughout the programme.[190] Historically, I don't think we should be debating exactly how much cancer, and how many deaths were prevented by the screening programme. The exact numbers depend on agreeing what would have happened in the absence of screening and in the presence of an epidemic of HPV infection that is very difficult to determine accurately. Nevertheless, we all agree that there were substantial numbers and the UK screening programme became among the best in the world; it was as effective as any other, I think, and probably more cost-effective than most.

Patrick Walker: There were important collaborations and publications in the 1990s. The first were by Ian Duncan in 1992 and 1997 with the publication of *Guidelines for Clinical Practice and Programme Management,* which brought together cytologists and colposcopists, and then David Luesley's publication, *Standards and Quality in Colposcopy,* which for the first time started to give some evidence base to the quality of care.[191] I think the other important thing about that time is that the programme became more woman-centred.[192] It was realized

[189] For details of the ICRF committee members, see note 51; ICRF Coordinating Committee on Cervical Screening (1986); see also Sasieni *et al.* (1996).

[190] NHS CSP (1996).

[191] See notes 60 and 63. See also Luesley (ed.) (1996).

[192] Marteau *et al.* (1990).

for the first time that a lot of unnecessary anxieties were experienced by women involved in the screening programme.

Gray: I was actually going to touch upon the question of the anxiety. It played a very big part in the public perception of the screening programme, and in the way the press reported aspects of the screening programme. Anxiety was heightened by the increase in litigation that took place as we started looking back at smears and found that abnormalities had been missed.[193] Lawyers became well aware that they could actually get very successful compensation through the courts. This whole aspect, I think, should be recorded as part of the history of the programme in the late 1980s and early 1990s. It had quite an impact on laboratories and on women.

McCluggage: It's something I have thought about with the National Cervical Cancer Audit, looking back at all cancers, the potential for more litigation coming out of this. Is this something that we are going to be faced with?

Sasieni: There are different views. I think there is going to be more litigation generally. But there are two audit activities going on. One is that any woman who gets cervical cancer, and even breast cancer, is entitled to know everything about her screening history, and that's been mandated by the Minister, so that's the one that could potentially be used for litigation.

I wanted to say two things historically. One is how the improvement in quality assurance led to more bad stories about cervical screening, and in the 1990s it seemed that every six months there was another story about a doctor taking a smear with his finger and about a lab that binned all the results. These things were happening because they had been happening for years and now they were being discovered.[194] Quality assurance put a stop to those bad practices, you don't get such stories very often nowadays. The other media-type issue, I am not so certain it was in the 1990s – Dr Szarewski could correct me – but the *Coronation Street* story, in terms of wanting to know what can be done with publicity, when Alma got cervical cancer, there was an increase in smears taken.[195] In all these poster campaigns and other campaigns that many PCTs

---

[193] Wilson (2000); see also Bryder (2008).

[194] See, for example, BBC News, UK Health: Thousands call cancer scare hotline, Wednesday, July 29, 1998 Published at 17:03 GMT 18:03, freely available at http://news.bbc.co.uk/1/hi/health/141391.stm (visited 6 October 2009).

[195] Alma Halliwell, a character in the television soap opera, was diagnosed with cervical cancer in June 2001 and died six weeks later. See Howe *et al.* (2002); Richardson *et al.* (2002).

did, no-one ever monitored any detectable effect on screening uptake. The invitations had a huge effect on coverage, but the only publicity about screening which had been shown to have an impact was the Alma episode.

Szarewski: It was a double-edged sword this, because we spent all of our time trying to make women less anxious about going for cervical screening. But, as Peter has said, the single most effective intervention in getting women to turn up for smears was the death of Alma in *Coronation Street*, which scared women out of their wits and attendance at screening shot up. It was written up in the *BMJ* and they concluded that it there was a demonstrable effect of that massive increase in anxiety caused by Alma's death.[196] In fact, the whole Alma story was extremely poorly done, because it actually couldn't have been attributed to a failure of screening. But nevertheless, all of that went by the board, the women were scared stiff and turned up.

McCluggage: We are going to move on to later developments and applying understanding of HPV.

Cubie: We started to talk earlier about some of the molecular techniques that had been developed in the 1980s and used in basic science and research situations. It's still a jump to think of using tests and technology in a clinical situation and that had to wait a little bit longer. I think we owe quite a lot to someone who isn't here, Attila Lörincz, who in the early 1990s was developing HPV hybridization methods that could be applied to clinical samples, both to sections and to smears.[197] Attila very kindly shared his HPV protocols in 1984/5, so I am not sure when he started doing this on clinical material, and I certainly went down the route of *in situ* hybridization for a while, because I am a diagnostic virologist, and basically we do cytology too. The difference was that we were looking for proteins in other viruses, and that's not so different from looking for the nucleic acid of specific viruses by *in situ* hybridization. There were things coming together in the early 1980s which linked virology and pathology but also led to developments in tests that could be suitable for diagnostic situations. The *in situ* hybridization unfortunately was not sensitive enough and perhaps put a lot of our gynaecologist colleagues off the results that could be obtained from mass HPV testing. Attila worked to produce the hybrid capture assays that have been used widely in recent years in studies around

---

[196] Howe *et al.* (2003).

[197] See, for example, Lörincz *et al.* (1986).

the world.[198] Actually, the technology for the hybrid capture assay is very good technology. It's a hybridization system that detects nucleic acid by amplifying the detection signal rather than the molecular tests we all hear about every day, polymerase chain reaction (PCR), which amplifies the nucleic acid directly. So, I guess hybrid capture first hit the market in the late 1980s, version 1 (HC-I), which was not that sensitive, but actually probably clinically quite relevant, because we then worked out that you could have a test that was too sensitive if you were trying to relate it to clinical needs.[199] That moved on to hybrid capture version 2 (HC-II), which everyone knows of or has read studies about.[200] I guess the first randomized controlled trial using HC-II in the UK was the 'HPV in addition to routine testing' (HART) study, which Jack Cuzick set up with Anne Szarewski – I was involved as were others – that was reported in 2003 in the *Lancet*.[201] In parallel with hybrid capture, other people were developing the PCR technique, particularly Jan Walboomers in the Amsterdam lab, and his colleague may talk more about this. They linked the PCR to a hybridization system which allowed them to type the virus. Those typing systems went beyond the screening possibilities of the hybrid capture assay and have given us tools that have been adapted by lots of companies, with commercial interest in competition now being fierce for different technologies, but that's in the last decade, not before 2000.

Peto: A technical point on hybrid capture: it does have a false positive rate, something between 1–3 per cent. This is quite a serious problem in older women, because in older women the prevalence of HPV is only a few per cent. It's a technical problem that still needs sorting out.

McCluggage: For those of us who don't know, does HC-II pick up all HPV types?

Peto: It picks up all types. All the ones that matter.

Cubie: It's a screening test. It uses a pool of probes which cover many high-risk genital types, and Julian is right to say that there is some cross-reactivity. It is not a false positive result though: these results are real HPV detection results, they are just not so clinically relevant. But a screening test – whether it

---

198 See, for example, Castle *et al.* (2003); Cope *et al.* (1997).

199 Clavel *et al.* (1998).

200 See Glossary, page 148; (2003); also note 216.

201 Cuzick *et al.* (2003).

is cytology, HPV, breast screening – will never be completely effective. You will always have an element of assessing sensitivity versus specificity, which is why it is very useful to have a range of other tests that allow us to go further and look at specific types of HPV. This happens in virology all the time – there's a difference between a screening test and a diagnostic test – and whatever we do, we usually have both available.

Jenkins: I think one of the important messages is that you can't really over-estimate the impact of HC-II in this field, can you? It's had such a huge impact, not just in the US where it was introduced, but in the UK and globally, and I think, perhaps, its major contribution in many ways is bringing HPV into the market place and then bringing it out into public awareness, particularly through some of the rather aggressive marketing techniques that are being used.[202] It is one of the ways in which HPV has been brought to the attention of the general public and I think these are important historical contributions, whereas the other testing systems have tended to remain much more research-based, much more restricted to the laboratories and to the experts.

Duncan: With regard to HPV testing, perhaps its greatest contribution has not actually been put into practice yet, and that is the negative predictive value, because if you are cytologically negative and you are HPV-negative, then you really are negative. Now, that allows us to discharge older women, who are never going to develop cervical cancer, from the screening programme early. And that's another aspect of the screening, because we at Dundee and Aberdeen have argued that it's unethical to subject women to screening if they are not at any significant risk.[203]

Wolfendale: A very quick comment. You say older women don't need screening. What about those who have new partners?

Duncan: It's all about fertile fields and in the older woman the cervix has matured. We wondered about the question of hormone replacement therapy and whether it would rejuvenate the cervix and create a transformation zone

---

[202] Professor David Jenkins wrote: 'One of the main methods used was direct-to-consumer advertising in journals and television, as is allowed in the US, aimed at focusing women's attention on sexually acquired HPV infection as an issue, encouraging women to ask for HPV testing at a clinic and to seek this additional test for extra reassurance about freedom of risk from cervical cancer. This was combined with active promotion among doctors in many countries at a time when the evidence remained inconclusive.' Note on draft transcript, 11 September 2009.

[203] Duncan (2004).

again, but that does not appear to be the case. The cervix has matured and is no longer the fertile ground for malignant transformation.

[Professor Valerie Beral reiterated the point that older women with new partners could be at risk.][204]

Jenkins: Can I make one comment here before we go off on to what is still a very active debate and certainly one which those of us who have been involved a lot in vaccination have to face almost every time we have to speak at any meeting. One intriguing issue is that we are only beginning to disclose the extent of natural protection against HPV in women who have successfully cleared an infection 30 years after the basic story of HPV was defined.[205] We are still a long way from answering some of these key questions.

Duncan: In the same population, we kept publishing the number of cases of CIN that we would have failed to detect if we had stopped screening women at the age of 50. And that's without HPV testing. I think that if HPV testing were brought in above the age of 35, in conjunction with cytology, this would allow us to reduce the frequency of screening and stop earlier.

Szarewski: Scotland, of course, is a more Presbyterian society perhaps, and it may be that sexual activity is less frequent there, but I think when we are talking about new partners, with respect to Margaret Wolfendale's question, I think we should mention that it's more likely that the 55-year-old man decides to have a younger female partner, and, because he feels obliged to have sex occasionally with his wife, he passes on the HPV from the younger partner he's having on the side to his older wife, who knows nothing about it for several years.

Peto: A point on the natural history: up to the age of *c.* 45 or 50, the probability of finding CIN2 or CIN3 is pretty much the same; if you detect HPV, it is lower above the age of 50. It depends what you mean by older women.

Sasieni: On the natural history: all the models looking at the time from CIN3 to progression of cancer showed that CIN3 is more likely to progress in older women, and the older you get the more likely it is to progress. I suspect that is because it's been persistent longer, and it's the persistent CIN3 that's most likely to progress. The importance of CIN3 in a woman in her fifties is probably much greater than the importance of CIN3 in a woman in her twenties.

---

[204] See also discussion on page 33.

[205] Jenkins (2006).

Herbert: But what about women of 65 who are HPV-positive? Do they go on being screened for ever? If they are positive and cytology is negative, what happens to them?

Cuzick: There are a lot of cancers found in women over the age of 65; it is still a major unmet need. So, I think we need to be very cautious about dropping off screening too early, when there are so many cancers still occurring in these older women, and we are doing very little about it.

Peto: HPV testing really does solve an awful lot of problems, particularly in older women where a lot of abnormal smears have nothing to do with HPV or cervical cancer risk.

McCluggage: We are going to move on to talk about HPV testing in triage and screening.

Cuzick: Triage and screening is still a very active topic, so I will try to confine myself primarily to some historical comments, and I think much of the work in this area really owes a big debt to Albert Singer, who was one of the first to recognize the clinical potential of all of this early work, discovering that HPV is the cause of cervix cancer and looking for ways in which this could be used in a clinical context.[206] I have been fortunate to work with a number of his scholars, starting with Michael Campion, Tony Hollingworth and Anne Szarewski (who is here today), on a range of studies, going back to the first study with Michael Campion in which it was found that women with low-grade smears that were HPV16-positive were more likely to have CIN3 on biopsy.[207] In retrospect, I think that was done with very old technology, before we had PCR, before we had hybrid capture, low specified dot blots, and probably one of the reasons that study was so successful was there was a lot of cross-hybridization. HPV16 detection would then be associated with all of these other types. Probably those early tests cross-hybridized with many different other high-risk types.[208]

I think the field has very much benefited from improvements in technologies as we have moved on. With PCR and hybrid capture and discoveries from some of the studies, we have moved away from the triage concept of this work (originally done with the Campion studies) and begun to move forward, to think: 'Can

---

206 See, for example, Campion *et al.* (1988); Mould *et al.* (2000).

207 Campion *et al.* (1986).

208 Professor Jack Cuzick wrote: 'High-risk HPV types are now thought to include 16, 18, 31, 35, 39, 45, 51, 52, 58 and 68.' Note on draft transcript, 4 September 2009.

this really be used in primary screening?' The first study of screening in normal-risk women with HPV, was the Margaret Pyke study, and again it was early technology. We screened for only four types (HPV16, -18, -31, and -33) and again were surprised at the first clear evidence that a lot of women were actually harbouring high-grade lesions that were negative on cytology.[209] The only way we found out about it was to have another test that was positive that led to a colposcopy. That was the first indication that cytology was not as good as we had thought, because we had another test which was actually saying we needed to do colposcopy as well. That moved on then to a larger study in older women, the Hammersmith study, then the multi-centre HART study.[210] So it's still a very, very active area. We still don't have HPV-introduced testing, even in triage, although I think the evidence for that is overwhelming. But if we are looking historically, I think a lot of that came out of the early work of Albert Singer.

McCluggage: This story seems to have been going on for an awfully long time now, this argument for HPV testing in the cervical screening programme. Is some decision going to be made in the near future, or what is happening at the moment?

Cuzick: I am probably the last one to answer that, because I spent ten years trying to get HPV considered for primary screening, and yet it is still a research question. I am also perplexed by the fact that we have been so slow to take this forward. I think it is a finding of major importance, and we do need to take these new technologies and evaluate them thoroughly, but not slowly; we need to be moving much more quickly on this. Again, cytology was a little bit its own worst enemy to some extent. Clearly cytology was a good screening test, and it did a substantial amount of good, and we must fully acknowledge that, but sometimes, we do need to move on. It is an old technology and there probably are better ways of doing what cytology is able to achieve.[211] I think that has been a difficult issue. We have something that works pretty darn well, but can we improve it with something that works a lot better? That's always a hard sell.

Smith: Mr Chairman, I think I can partly answer your question. The NHS Cervical Screening Programme (CSP) has recently instituted what is known as sentinel sites, of which there are six sites in England, including my own

---

[209] Cuzick *et al.* (1995).

[210] Cuzick *et al.* (2008); Cuzick *et al.*, (HART) (2003).

[211] See for example, Schiffman and Castle (2006).

laboratory, the Sheffield Cervical Cytology Service.[212] There they are looking at practical implementation of HPV testing for triage of low-grade abnormality and test of cure and that study commenced a few months ago.

McCluggage: So this was triage of what?

Smith: Low-grade abnormalities.

Jenkins: So why was the decision taken to have sentinel sites rather than to implement triage?

Smith: It is a pilot to look at the practical implementation, particularly the relationship of HPV with cytology.

Herbert: Can I say something about poor old cytology here? Most of the places that are implementing clinical trials of HPV as a primary screening test are using cytology triage. They still need cytology – because HPV may indicate a risk of CIN in the future, but cytology shows that an abnormality is present now. So, they do still need us; we don't need to hand in our resignations yet.

Sasieni: To try to answer the question about 'why' they are operating sentinel sites rather than rolling it out nationwide. I was on the advisory committee looking at the results from the three primary pilots, two of which looked at HPV triage, and the results were not as clearcut as in the research studies.[213] There was a big question as to who was going to pay for the HPV testing. The Department of Health was saying: 'There's no extra money, the screening programme already costs us £170 million a year or something in that region, and that's it'. It was Henry Kitchener's idea,[214] I think, to get a little bit of money in order to be able to do triage, continuing in the pilot sites and add Manchester and Liverpool. To make sure that it continued, everyone agreed that HPV triage

---

[212] The NHS CSP introduced HPV sentinel sites at six laboratories in autumn 2007 at Bristol, Northwick Park (Harrow), Liverpool, Manchester, Norwich and Sheffield. See www.cancerscreening.nhs.uk/cervical/hpv-sentinel-sites.html (visited 22 July 2009).

[213] See Legood *et al.* (2006); Moss *et al.* (Liquid-based Cytology/Human Papillomavirus Cervical Pilot Studies Group) (2006).

[214] Professor Henry Kitchener, Manchester, led a trial in 2001 to investigate HPV as a primary screening test funded by the Health Technology Assessment (HTA) programme, at Manchester, Stockport, Wigan and Leigh and Salford and Trafford (Sargent *et al.* (2008)). The Medical Research Council (MRC) and NHS in England and Scotland funded 'Trial of Management of Borderline and Other Low Grade Abnormal smears' (TOMBOLA) study, headed by Professor Norman Waugh, which began in 1999. See Patnick (ed.) (2008a); see also note 228.

shouldn't stop, it needed to be rolled out in a much more controlled fashion, because the results were disappointing, and it was fairly easy to get enough money to do HPV triage in just five sites.

McCluggage: What about the experiences in other countries? Is there anything that we can learn from those? Has it been successful in other countries?

Miller: There's a randomized trial ongoing in Finland. Matti Hakama has been very successful in arranging to evaluate new technology in a randomized fashion and the preliminary results seem to suggest that the peak difficulties are the specificity, the sensitivity in relation to the cytology is not greatly superior.[215] He is beginning to look at the question of changing the relative light units (RLU) cut-off level,[216] raising the level at which you declare a positive, and believes that in doing that he can achieve with HPV testing the relevant specificity associated with cytology. In British Columbia the decision has been taken to run a trial that has been initiated, comparing HPV testing every four years with a safety net of two years in another group with the two-year cytology, which is their standard. That trial has only just started; I don't think there's going to be much reported on it for a while.

Singer: Historically, as clinicians, we recognized probably about eight or nine years ago the enormous value of a negative HPV result with the negative predictive value in many trials being 99 per cent.[217] Approximately 5–7 per cent of all women in this country have a borderline smear. In the US they have used it as a reflex test in women with a borderline smear or 'atypical squamous cells of undetermined significance' (ASC-US, the US equivalent[218]), and saved an enormous amount of money by excluding women with a negative test. But, more importantly, the anxiety of women patients is reduced and a negative result really does mean negative.

---

[215] Anttila *et al.* (2006); Kotaniemi-Talonen *et al.* (2008a).

[216] Testing for HPV DNA with HC-II is a molecular biological method that tests for the presence of HPV DNA through a chemoluminescent reaction based on hybridization. Viral presence is measured in relative light units and reported as a ratio of relative light units (rlu ratio), a measure of luminescence. Samples with a ratio of less than 1.0 are classified as negative for high-risk HPV DNA and those 1.0 or above are positive. See Kotaniemi-Talonen *et al.* (2008b); Peyton *et al.* (1998).

[217] Wright *et al.* (2004).

[218] ASC-US is a classification of squamous intraepithelial lesions. For a discussion of UK and US grading, see Slater *et al.* (2005).

Cubie: Professor Sasieni asked: 'Who's going to pay?' Doesn't that sound familiar? Isn't that what most of this story of cervical screening has been about? And how cytology started? Who's going to pay? People did not know how they would fund screening, but started getting on with it. And, what has been achieved since 1988 is but a series of tweaks, which are the things which Tony Miller was talking about, the tweaks which will need to be put in place once we actually get down to it.

Sasieni: What is going on in other places? HPV in triage of borderline or, as the Americans call it, ASC-US cytology, is routine in North America, I think, and is used elsewhere. There's a new, fast HPV test, which is a hybrid capture test, for developing countries, which I believe is going to be adopted as the primary screening test in Colombia.[219] So there is more HPV testing going on elsewhere. In addition to the randomized trial in Finland, there are randomized trials in Italy, Sweden and the Netherlands, and all four of them show higher sensitivity for the detection of high-grade CIN on the first round, and those that have published second-round results show lower detection of high grade CIN in the HPV arm on the second round.[220] Yes, more women will be sent to colposcopy. The Finns have a very negative interpretation of the results, but their results are pretty much the same as others, and the Italians have a very positive interpretation of the same sort of results.

Szarewski: I think the problem with the HPV testing is the specificity to which we have alluded. The trouble is that although we keep talking about how wonderful it is to have a negative HPV test, in the pilot studies of triage in the UK, it made no difference to the women themselves. When looking at the anxiety levels in women with borderline smears and a negative HPV test, it made no difference, because they didn't understand what it meant. So if we are going to introduce HPV testing, which I do think is inevitable eventually, we mustn't forget the real importance of education of the public, because otherwise it's wasted. The patients are as anxious with a negative HPV test and a borderline smear as they would have been with the borderline smear, or even, in fact, a positive HPV test. What, then, is the point in doing it?

Professor Leslie Walker: To put this in historical perspective, in the 1970s and 1980s there was increasing interest in the psychosocial aspect of the diagnosis

---

[219] See, for example, WHO (2002).

[220] Ronco *et al.*, New Technologies for Cervical Cancer Working Group (2006, 2008); Mayrand *et al.*, Canadian Cervical Cancer Screening Trial Study Group (2007); Kotaniemi-Talonen *et al.* (2008a and b); Naucler *et al.* (2007); Bulkmans *et al.* (2007).

and the treatment of cancer, particularly in the disciplines of nursing, psychology and psychiatry. In the early 1980s, when the British Psychosocial Oncology Society was founded, I think it is fair to say that initial interest focused on what one might call 'screening distress', the effect of getting an abnormal smear result.[221] One of the early studies by Beresford and Gervaize showed that all of the women that they surveyed were afraid that they would have cancer.[222] Many – two-thirds – were afraid of the medical procedures involved in the investigation, and this fear showed itself in a range of behavioural changes, including sleep disturbance, irritability, relationship difficulties, including problems with sexual relationships. It was also clear even then that there were other issues for these women, including uncertainty about fertility and the possibility of transmission of disease to their partners.

The second area of interest was investigational and procedural distress. Some studies showed that anticipatory anxiety was similar, or equal to, that produced by some types of surgery.[223] Also, Campion and colleagues showed that, compared with a comparison group of women, six months after colposcopy, biopsy and laser vaporization, women had less sexual interest, less frequency of intercourse and more negative feelings towards their partners.[224]

People have studied several ways of attempting to ameliorate this distress, particularly leaflets and booklets, and these have generally been of some help, but not for all women.[225] Counselling has also been investigated, although there aren't many studies.[226] Women usually say that it's helpful, but interestingly, most studies show that there's no significant effect on objective measures of health-related quality of life.

Then there's the issue of gynaecological intervention for an abnormal smear, for example, the effects of 'see and treat' versus surveillance and, indeed, this is how my interest in this field was stimulated. Stephen Bell and colleagues in Aberdeen had shown that colposcopy was associated with persistent anxiety

---

[221] For further details, see www.bpos.org/ (visited 29 April 2009).

[222] Beresford and Gervaize (1986).

[223] Rogstad (2002): particularly page 365.

[224] Campion *et al.* (1988).

[225] See, for example, www.womens-health.co.uk/smear.asp; www.womenshealthlondon.org.uk/leaflets/cervical/cervab.html; www.bbc.co.uk/health/womens_health/issues_smeartest.shtml (visited 29 April 2009).

[226] See, for example, Wolfe *et al.* (1992).

following surveillance, but it wasn't a randomized trial.[227] He came to see me subsequently to seek advice on how to validate screening tests for clinically significant anxiety and depression in a further study.

In 1998 I was very pleased to be invited by Julian Little to lead on the psychosocial aspects of a randomized controlled trial subsequently funded by the MRC (TOMBOLA).[228] This was a study of over 4000 women from Grampian, Tayside and Nottingham, who had low-grade abnormal cytology and were randomized either to cytological surveillance in primary care or to colposcopy. Compared with surveillance, colposcopy was associated with less clinically significant anxiety in the short term. However, in the longer term, there was no difference in the levels of anxiety or depression between these management policies. But, more specifically, women managed by surveillance were more worried about the next smear being positive; they were more worried generally about their health; and they were more worried about whether they could have children in the future.

Turning to the issue of HPV specifically, McCaffery *et al.* showed, and we have already heard a little bit about this, that women who were HPV-positive were more anxious and felt more worried about sexual relationships than those who were HPV-negative, regardless of whether their smears were normal or abnormal.[229]

Finally, there is the issue of non-participation in the screening programme. Again, we have heard something about this. But in addition to socio-demographic factors and ethnicity, there are a number of clinic-specific factors and psychological factors which seem to be related to this. For example, non-participation is associated with having a fear of cancer, not having a female cytoscreener available, a worry about embarrassment and pain, the belief that screening is not going to be of any benefit and the perception of being at low risk of cervical cancer.

So, to conclude, over the last 20 years or so, people have become increasingly aware that there is a personal cost and a psychosocial cost to cervical screening, and more recently to HPV testing also. And clearly there is a continuing need to develop ways to minimize that, and to encourage current non-participants to attend for screening.

---

[227] Bell *et al.* (1995).

[228] For further details, see Cotton *et al.* (2006).

[229] McCaffery *et al.* (2004).

Szarewski: I am conscious that I am slipping beyond 2000 by saying this, but coming back to the education aspect, I think it's ironic that the advent of the HPV vaccines is providing an absolutely fantastic platform for educating the public about HPV in general, because the press are really interested in the vaccines, which they have never been in any other aspect of HPV.[230] So ironically, the vaccines are providing us with the opportunity to educate everybody about HPV in general.

Singer: We know as a result of the vaccine and doing many pre-introduction interviews in the form of an online questionnaire survey, which showed that a substantial amount of ignorance was present at all levels, extending from the administrators in the government all the way down to the actual women, mothers, etc.[231] The most important thing now is to get knowledge of HPV passed on to all of them.

Mr Patrick Walker: Not to put too much of a down note on it, what we have been looking at over the last three or four hours is the enormous success of a population-based screening programme that came out of a disorganized and under-funded programme. The keys for success that we have seen are a consistent level of public investment in the organization of the programme, and the high coverage of the population at risk. For all of the great opportunities that vaccination offers for the 12- and 13-year-old women, partial implementation of the vaccine programme, which doesn't have all of the viral types in a catch-up group, might lead to false assurance of young vaccinated women who are still at risk of the disease, reduced compliance with the programme, and reduced coverage. Ironically, this could undermine the success of the programme we have now, particularly if the cash-strapped primary care trusts having to invest in the organization, particularly of the catch-up programme, are tempted to reduce the budget that currently goes towards screening quality assurance.

Peto: The amount of money spent on the vaccine will be almost as much as on the screening programme, and we'll have to go on screening as well until a polyvalent vaccine against all the common HPV types is available and affordable.[232] Western

---

[230] See, for example, Chan and Berek (2007); FUTURE II Study Group (2007).

[231] Sherris *et al.* (2006).

[232] For an economic evaluation of the two vaccines currently in use in the UK, see Jit *et al.* (2008): a769; and other perspectives, see Franco *et al.* (2006). For estimates of the cost of screening compared with the cost of a life saved, see Bryant and Stevens (1995); Waugh and Robertson (1996); Waugh *et al.* (1996a and b); Peto *et al.* (2004a) and note 158.

governments should be collaborating to develop a cheap polyvalent vaccine as rapidly as possible. That would save them hundreds of millions of pounds, and would also prevent cervical cancer in developing countries where most of the cases and deaths occur and where effective screening isn't viable.

Jenkins: I feel I have to say something on this, because that really is a gross oversimplification of what's quite a complex development of vaccines, and the issue of multivalent and polyvalent vaccines is unfortunately not as simple as you would have us believe in that impassioned speech. I think if it were simple to generate these polyvalent vaccines, then it would have been done, and certainly both the vaccine companies are working on these currently.[233] However, this is all going well beyond 2000, we are now looking at probably 2010, 2011, 2012, before any of these become anything like the possibility of reality, and we have to work with what we have got. Having said that, it is the ultimate goal; there's no question that things will continue to develop beyond what we have now. If I can get back to the point that Anne Szarewski was making, I think one of the huge impacts of the vaccine, apart from its potential clinical benefits, has been that it has opened up HPV to the world in general, and meant that we are not a small community of eccentrics exploring a rather exotic virus that most people have never even heard about.

Sasieni: To return to the personal, the screening programme in England – it may have been after 2000 – started this new information, informed choice. But there has certainly been a huge debate, some of it by Professor Peto, even more passionate than he has been today, about the information that should be provided. There were individuals whom I won't mention by name, who seemed to emphasize the downside of screening the whole time, and were accused, I think, of causing the deaths of thousands of women by putting them off going for screening.[234] Then there are people who felt that actually virtually all you needed to do was to promote the positive side of screening. There was a general agreement over time that we try to get a more balanced approach to the information, although it's always very difficult because there is no agreement among the experts about what is a balanced approach to the information. Certainly, there was a huge change from 1988 until 1999, in terms of the attitude of providing information and the general feeling in society that the

---

[233] Professor David Jenkins wrote: 'The two companies currently working on a polyvalent vaccine for HPV are GSK and Merck.' Comment on draft transcript, 11 August 2009.

[234] Raffle *et al.* (2003); listen to Dr Angela Raffle and Mrs Julietta Patnick discussing changes in cervical screening on Woman's Hour, 22 October 2003, at: www.bbc.co.uk/radio4/womanshour/2003_42_wed_02.shtml (visited 4 September 2009).

medical profession should be less paternalistic. Women needed to be told the downside of screening, even it if puts them off attending.

Campo: Three comments: the first is that the vaccine is type-specific, and one thing that has, in my mind, not been extensively investigated is that L2 protein should have been incorporated in the vaccine. It induces cross-reactive neutralizing antibodies, but it's not there. It's something that should be thought about. The second thing is that it is not quite so easy in terms of adding VLPs to the vaccine, because these are, surely, different HPV types, with a different incidence in different parts of the world. So while HPV16 and HPV18 are global, HPV58 is in Hong Kong but not in Brazil; and so on and so forth. If you want to add more and more VLPs I think we should start adding them differentially to the vaccine from Brazil, and the vaccine for Hong Kong, and I don't think anybody is going to do that. My third comment is about education. Professor Sasieni said that people should be educated from the administrators down, and this is my own experience, that even doctors do not understand what the current vaccine is about. Treating CIN2 with the current vaccine is like throwing money down the drain; clearly there are doctors who do not know what the vaccine can do. The vaccine is fantastic, but it has to be used properly.

Jenkins: I am very glad that everybody is discussing the vaccine, but we really have to limit discussion on that at the moment. Certainly, the L2 vaccine has been looked at. There are some issues around that; there is some recent work that suggests perhaps some of the differences, geographical differences, that are claimed in HPV types may not be as great as they appear to be and that some of this is due to very small studies in very special populations. Like the HPV58 in Hong Kong, it is based on very small numbers.

Singer: We could only dream about the vaccine. There was an editorial from 23 years ago in the *British Journal of Obstetrics and Gynaecology* by Dennis McCance and myself, talking about the association of HPV and cervical cancer and we weren't sure whether the association was causal or casual. We said that the most satisfactory evidence or proof would be if a vaccine were produced against HPV in the future, which would show a reduction in the vaccinated women at greatest risk. This, we said, would be a difficult task.[235] Thankfully, in the end it wasn't as impossible as we thought it would be.

---

[235] Singer and McCance wrote: 'The association of HPV infections and neoplasias of the lower genital tract, but is this association causal or casual? The most satisfactory evidence would be if a vaccine were produced against HPVs and show a reduction in the vaccinated women at greatest risk. This will be a difficult task' (Singer and McCance (1985): 1085).

McCluggage: Very true words. It remains for me to say that this has been a very successful Witness Seminar and Dr Tansey will speak after I have finished. I would like to thank all the audience for their participation. I have enjoyed this very much and, as a non-HPV person, I have learned a lot, and I hope everybody else has and has enjoyed the Witness Seminar.

Tansey: Yes, I would like to thank you all very much for coming. It's been a very interesting, educational, informative, and at times very amusing and entertaining afternoon. I also have learned an awful lot. As I mentioned at the beginning, this meeting is the tip of the iceberg. We will now translate the transcript of this Witness Seminar into readable text and we shall need your help in doing that. On your way home tonight, many of you will think: 'Oh why didn't I say so and so?' You will have the opportunity of putting that into the transcript at a later date as a footnote. If you have any papers or references you would like us to have or that we could copy, please get in touch with us and let us know.

I would like to offer the thanks of the History of Twentieth Century Medicine Group to David Jenkins, whose idea this was originally, and who has worked very closely with Lois Reynolds, Wendy Kutner and myself in planning this, and also thank Lois and Wendy for all their hard work in rushing around with the microphones, and especially to Glenn, whose timing of this meeting has meant that we have finished right on the dot, and to invite you all to have a glass of wine.

Appendix 1

The emergence of the natural history of cervical cancer

Professor Leopold G Koss
Montefiore Medical Center and Albert Einstein College of Medicine, Bronx, New York, NY

In 1842, an Italian physician, Domenico Rigoni-Stern, published a series of mortality statistics of women dying of cancer in the city of Verona.[236] In this first epidemiological analysis, Rigoni-Stern pointed out that 'cancer of the uterus' was much more common in married women and widows than in virgins and nuns. This was the first suggestion that 'cancer of the uterus' was somehow related to sexual activity. It may be safely assumed that most of the women in Verona died of cancer of the uterine cervix because that was, at that time and remained for over 100 years, the most common form of cancer of the female genital tract. In spite of many speculations, the nature of the sexually transmitted cancerous agent remained a mystery.

The concept that cancer of the uterine cervix was preceded by precancerous states limited to the epithelium must be attributed to a 1908 paper by an Austrian gynaecologist, Walther Schauenstein.[237] This concept was essential for cervix cancer prevention programmes which were based on recognition and elimination of precancerous states, thus preventing invasive cancer.

Cytologic screening became one method of recognition of precancerous states. Although the method is attributed to George Papanicolaou, who presented a paper on the use of vaginal smears in detection of uterine cancer in 1928,[238] he had a predecessor, a Romanian pathologist, Aureli Babeş, who published a beautifully illustrated paper on this topic in the French publication, *Presse Medicale*, prior to Papanicolaou's presentation.[239] Babeş, using direct cervical samples, proposed that cancer of the cervix can be recognized in preinvasive stages. Papanicolaou's primary interest was the sequence of events in the menstrual cycle which he could study by means of vaginal smears. He did not pursue his

---

[236] Rigoni-Stern (1842). See also note 85.

[237] Schauenstein (1908).

[238] Papanicolaou (1928).

[239] Babeş (1928); see also note 4.

observations on cancer for ten years, for lack of access to clinical material, until a fortuitous association with the gynaecologist, Herbert Traut, in 1938. Traut provided him with vaginal smears, the topic of the paper published in 1941.[240] This was the beginning of the 'Pap smear.' Papanicolaou never acknowledged Babeş' contribution. It is alleged that this omission cost him a Nobel award.

Direct sampling of the uterine cervix was rediscovered by a Canadian gynaecologist/cytologist, J Ernest Ayre in 1949.[241] Among the many varieties of cells observed in the cervical smears, there were some that were characterized by large nuclei and large, clear perinuclear spaces. These cells were extensively studied by Ayre, who called them 'halo cells' and considered them to be precursors of cervical cancer.[242] In 1960, Ayre proposed that the 'halo cells' may represent a viral manifestation in premalignancy.[243]

The term, koilocytes, in common use today to describe these cells, was derived from the term 'koilocytotic atypia' proposed by Koss and Durfee in 1956.[244] The term reflected the hollow nature of the clear perinuclear space (Greek: koilos = cavity, kytos = cell). The histologic equivalent of koilocytes was named 'warty atypia' because of its resemblance to warts or condylomas. The suggestion that koilocytes were a specific manifestation of a viral infection became plausible with the recognition that genital condylomas were a sexually transmitted disease caused by a virus, as documented by Dunn and Ogilvie in 1968.[245] The cytologic similarity of condylomas to 'warty atypia' was noted in the first edition of my book in 1961.[246] In two synchronous papers, Meisels and Fortin from Canada and Purola and Savia from Finland proposed that the koilocytes may be a link to condylomas, hence the viral origin of cervical cancer.[247] The first documentation that the nuclei of koilocytes contained viral particles was

---

[240] Papanicolaou and Traut (1941).

[241] Ayre (1949).

[242] Ayre and Ayre (1949).

[243] Ayre (1960).

[244] Koss and Durfee (1956); see also Figure 4, page 35.

[245] Dunn and Ogilvie (1968).

[246] Koss (1961); see also note 98.

[247] Meisels and Fortin (1976); Purola and Savia (1977).

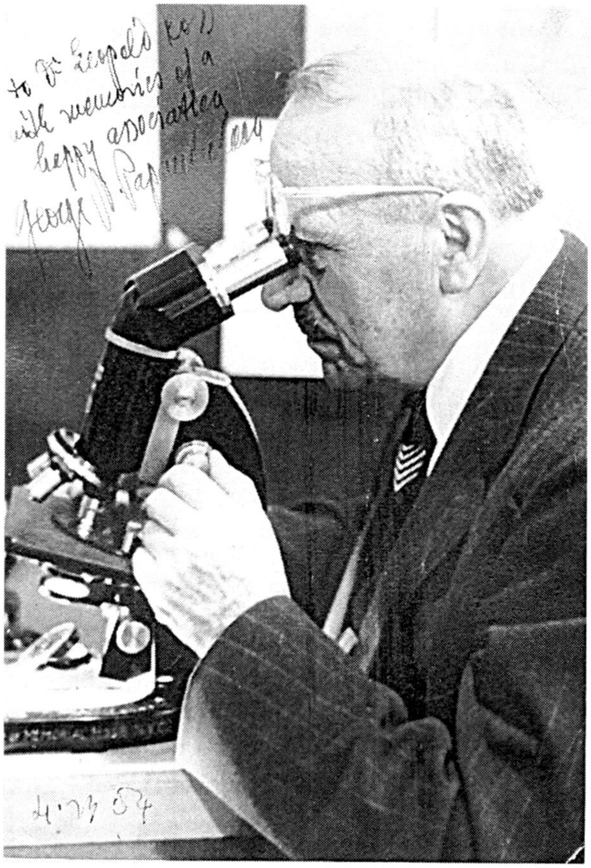

Figure 7: Dr George N Papanicolaou at the microscope.
Photo inscribed to Leopold G Koss on 23 April 1954.

presented by Laverty *et al.* from Australia in 1978.[248] Presumably, it is this work that generated the interest of virologists in papillomavirus in biopsies of the uterine cervix and the beginning of classification of viral types, as shown by zur Hausen and Gissmann.[249] There were many other contributors to this sequence of events that led to subclassification of human papillomaviruses into low-risk and high-risk types and to antiviral vaccines.

There are still many unanswered questions about the relationship of human papillomavirus to cervical cancer. The mechanism of viral penetration into

[248] Laverty *et al.* (1978).

[249] zur Hausen (1987); Gissmann and zur Hausen (1976).

the epithelium is not known. The reason why, among many young women infected with human papillomavirus, only a very few progress to cancer, is not understood, in keeping with the unpredictable behaviour of precancerous lesions of the cervix in a long-term follow-up study.[250] The possibility of one or more contributing factors explaining the relationship of viral infection to cancer still needs to be explored. Some of the remaining mysteries have to do with the presence of human papillomavirus in cancers of organs that are clearly not related to sexual activity, such as the cornea of the eye and the oesophagus, the latter particularly in China.[251]

I had the rare privilege of knowing Dr Papanicolaou and working with him. I also got to know personally most of the key participants in the sequence of events briefly summarized above, stretching over the past half a century.

Having read the text of the discussions that took place during the Witness Seminar, I realized that I know personally several of the participants and knew many whom have either died or are no longer active. In the UK, as in most other countries, cytological screening for cervical cancer was pioneered by gynecologists, because pathologists had no interest in processing the time-consuming and poorly rewarded Pap smears. Among the pathologists, there were a few notable exceptions: Herbert Fidler organized a screening programme in Vancouver, British Columbia; James Reagan of Cleveland and Stanley Patten of Rochester, New York, wrote extensively about the correlation between cell patterns and tissues in cervical material.

The true proponents of cervical screening in the US were gynaecologists and the first major book on the subject was written by a cytotechnologist, Ruth Graham.[252] Not surprisingly, the first American organization dealing with cytological diagnosis of cancer was named the Intersociety Cytology Council as it consisted of gynaecologists, cytologists and the few interested pathologists. Today, the organization is known as the American Society of Cytopathology. In the UK, the proponents of cytologic screening for cervical cancer were the gynaecologists, Stanley Way and Erica Wachtel. The latter was a refugee from Vienna, Austria, another gift from Mr Hitler to the civilized world. She was the mentor of Professor Dulcie Coleman. Nasseem Husain of London also played a

---

[250] Koss *et al.* (1963).

[251] For a summary, see Koss (1961).

[252] The second edition (Graham (1963)) of a volume originally published from the Vincent Memorial Hospital laboratory, Boston, published in 1950.

major role in these events. Although there is no doubt that Harald zur Hausen, the recent Nobel Prizewinner, and his co-workers were instrumental in the study of human papillomavirus as a factor in the genesis of carcinoma of the cervix, I have little doubt that this work was influenced by cytological observations that suggested a viral origin of cervical cancer. The story is more complicated than is generally assumed and it was a privilege to have participated in it in some way.

I can only repeat the words of Michel de Montaigne (1533–92):[253]

> It might well be said of me that in this book I have only made up a bunch of other men's flowers, providing of my own only the string that ties them together.

[253] Montaigne (1580).

Appendix 2

Reminiscences on cervical screening

From Dr Arthur Spriggs (written 12 September 2009)

I joined the pathology department at the Radcliffe Infirmary, Oxford. In the haematology department under Gwyn Macfarlane I began studying the cells of serous fluids, and started my DM thesis (1952) which became the basis of a monograph 'The cytology of effusions' (1957).[254] With a grant provided by Dr A H T Robb-Smith (pathology) and Professor John Chassar Moir (gynaecology), I spent three months in the US and Canada studying the cytology of vaginal and cervical smears using the Papanicolaou methods; 'cytodiagnosis' was usually practised independently of the department of morbid anatomy. So while learning from the leading cytologists, the variably sceptical opinions of the local histopathologists were also sought. On my return, with the assistance of Michael Boddington, I inaugurated the cytodiagnostic service in Oxford. At first this was for gynaecological outpatients, but in the 1960s was extended to screening of the local population. The expanding laboratory was transferred to the Churchill Hospital. Grants were provided by the British Empire Cancer Campaign (Cancer Research Campaign from 1970) for research into various aspects of cytological diagnosis – in particular, cyto-histological correlation in sputum and stomach washings, as well as cervical smears (1953–60); identification of tumour cells in circulating blood, also in cerebrospinal fluid (1959–61); and chromosomes of human malignant cells (1960–72). It became apparent that each malignant tumour was a new unique clone of cells with an altered chromosome complement. This was most easily demonstrated in the cells of effusions, but from a small number of biopsy fragments from the cervix when there was evidence of the same process in carcinoma *in situ*.[255] From the late 1960s, attempts were made to follow up cases in which a 'positive' cervical smear had escaped from further recommended procedures over at least two years. Some of these were found again, particularly with the collaboration of Professor Richard Doll's department, and a picture could be presented showing the proportion regressing or progressing over the years, evidently a positive smear

[254] Spriggs (1957).

[255] Spriggs *et al.* (1971).

is dangerous to ignore.[256] Concerning automated cytodiagnosis in the 1970s, the proposal which I thought achievable would be to pre-screen smears with a machine capable of marking any large or hyperchromatic nuclei, so that the screener could go at once to significant areas of the smear. We failed to achieve this with the apparatus then available. Before my retirement in 1984, collaborative studies were done with the histopathologists using immunochemical methods, some of which appeared promising in the identification of malignant cells in effusions. Following my retirement, I completed with M M Boddington a new fully illustrated book on the cytology of serious effusions.[257]

From Dr Nasseem Husain (written 2 April 2001, 16 and 31 May 2008)

I recognized the value of cytological screening both here and in many countries elsewhere in the world when I went on lecture tours in the US, South America, Europe, Asia and Japan to promote this concept. The need for a defined screening programme which was argued by me through the central committees of the Ministry of Health resulted in and the establishment of cytology screening units in every hospital and by general practitioners. In this I was aided and strongly supported by Marks and Spencers, whose medical staff I knew well and they were the first to create mobile screening units in this country, where around 7000 tests per year were carried out on their female employees on a two-to-three year recall, conducting field analysis of different techniques and follow-up programmes (1967–89). Many of the smears went to local laboratories, but M&S also provided a magnificent laboratory for me at St Stephen's Hospital along with the salaries of three technicians and half of a clerk and provided many other assets, where, as well as screening, we also looked at detailed morphology of chromatin patterns. Although many doctors took up the practice of cytology, few of them were histopathologist or haematologists and the practice sadly moved away from scientific cellular pathology and a separate specialty of cytology developed. (31 May 2008)

I was the first NHS consultant in cytopathology in the UK, being appointed in 1961, but was also very actively involved in the development of screening programmes, training of pathologists and technicians, development of automation techniques and in cytochemistry. (16 May 2008)

---

[256] Kinlen and Spriggs (1978).

[257] Spriggs and Boddington (1989). Excerpt from a letter to Dr Winifred Gray, 12 September 2009, which will be deposited with the other records of the meeting in archives and manuscripts, Wellcome Library, London, at GC/253.

I was involved in research and development of a non-wettable swab, plastic spatula and a more appropriately shaped knuckle-ended wooden spatula in the mid-1970s which has ultimately resulted in the Aylesbury spatula ten years later (see Figure 6, page 54).

Trials were undertaken of an irrigation cytopipette as a self-collecting instrument to identify its 75–80 per cent accuracy compared with the spatula, but at about one-fifth the cost, and the development of our own British model of the pipette, to my specifications and an improved irrigation and preservative solution and eventually, the greater acceptability as a screening procedure in a controlled trial supported by the Ministry of Health (DHSS after 1968).

The development of cell preparatory techniques for automated scanners utilizing cell dispersal systems of mucolytic, chemical, enzymic and physical methods, which include a study of ultrasonics, disaggregation by sheer stress techniques using syringes, vortex whistle, peristaltic pumps and cell 'spinners' on to film strips and glass slides. Research into the cell coatings from 90.000 to 500.000 molecular weight with a cell spread utilizable for any subsequent staining process and for use with cyst fluid, urine and fine needle aspirate samples.

An extensive study was made for use with automatic scanners to produce a high signal-to-noise ratio and achieve a machine-blind stain. This involved a review of a range of haematoxylins and DNA stains and the development of a quantitative fast gallocyanin of 5–10 minutes' duration, instead of the 18-hour schedule of Einarson (1932), to which cytoplasmic stains could be added.

In 1965, I evaluated the claim that the Coulter cell counter with a size distribution plotter would demonstrate secondary peaks of large cells in neoplastic cell samples. This was examined in a joint venture with the Royal Marsden Hospital to demonstrate that the large cell was in fact a cell cluster, probably polymorphs, and often in association with malignancy, but that these secondary peaks would disappear on cell cluster disaggregation.

In 1966 we were the first to explore the use of a static cell scanner by the conversion of the industrial Quantimet B imaging analysing computer using a Vidicon television tube from an incidental light microscope to a transmission light instrument. A study of cells from cervical smears demonstrated that there were sufficient discrete neoplastic cells stained by haematoxylin which were over-threshold, giving a raised integrated optical density, which could be registered by virtue of sizing and density potentiometers and be recalled for interactive visual assessment. These results were presented in the first automatic research conference in 1968. A purpose-built scanner called the Imaco cytoscreen was then constructed to my specifications and funded by the DHSS. This project led the international field in conferences in Europe and the US for the next five to ten years. The further development of this scanner failed to be adequately supported by the DHSS and subsequently by the MRC, as I had to transfer our energies to the Cervifip (Cytoscan 110), an offshoot of the metaphase finder and chromosome analyser being developed by the MRC, first in London and then at the Western General Hospital, Edinburgh, 1978–89. We were closely involved in perfecting this diode array scanner over the last five to ten years of my appointment, which resulted in a sophisticated instrument with a low false negative signal rate achieved by the register of aneuploid and polyploidy nuclei, with rejection of the false positive signals due to nuclear overlaps and cell debris, by pattern recognition, but has not yet reached acceptable limits. Nevertheless, this instrument compares well with the three to four instruments developed in Europe and the US and can read and sort cells at the rate of about 150 000 per two minutes.

I had considerable experience in flow cell instruments and our comparative trials using flow cell analysers and microdensitometers does demonstrate the unique advantage of our fast static cell scanner (Cervifip), working on both the rapid cell detection of the rare event and also on analyzing disaggregated selective archival material from tissue blocks in order to study the ploidy pattern of cells of tumours and therefore to relate to the prognostic and the therapeutic effects and able to achieve a valuable prospective dimension if fine needle aspirate samples are used.

The limitation of morphological criteria for the diagnosis of malignancy encourage me to pursue a study in depth of the biochemical and functional parameters of neoplastic cells and it is here that our researches embraced both biochemical and cytochemical fields. Our study of the glucose-6-phosphate dehydrogenase enzyme in vaginal aspirates was based on a claim of raised activity in neoplasia and a survey of some 5000 case samples tested against traditional scrape smear cytology to confirm or disprove this thesis resulted in the finding that although all invasive lesions showed high levels, only about half the carcinoma *in situ* cases did so and there was an excessively high proportion of false positive readings. It was later found that if potassium was used as a measure of cellular content and therefore the source of enzyme rather than freeze dried weight or cytochrome, the false positive rate dropped to less than 9 per cent. Such a test could conceivably be used to screen for endometrial cancer.

We were the first to study the state of the DNA in neoplasia by a slowed-down Feulgen hydrolysis technique at room temperature to show that there was a significant labile component, both in the neoplastic cell and also in the benign cells in their vicinity, a feature that may make the detection of malignancy possibly without encountering or identifying a neoplastic cell.

The combined output of the Charing Cross and St Stephen's cytology departments was about 55 000 tests per year. An increasing proportion of these were becoming non-gynaecological tests presenting a substantial workload in the fields of gastrointestinal and pulmonary brush specimens and fine needle aspirates. The gynaecological screening load used to come from a large area of south-west London and from parts of Sussex where we served about 55 different gynaecological screening clinics, 22 hospital clinics and about 130 general practitioners. On the transfer of the district to North West Thames Regional Health Board, the range of GPs and clinics was reduced but the volume of throughout dropped only marginally, while problem cervical smears and non-gynaecological specimens, including fine needle aspirates and AIDs specimens, increased markedly. (2 April 2001)

I must finally congratulate you on your initiative to choose this field of cytodiagnosis as a subject for a Witness Seminar, which has effectively spread to many other parts of the body and is now a highly sophisticated and effective method of early diagnosis. (31 May 2008)

References

Ahluwalia H S, Doll R. (1968) Mortality from cancer of the cervix uteri in British Columbia and other parts of Canada. *British Journal of Preventive and Social Medicine* **22**: 161–4.

Andermann A, Blancquaert I, Beauchamp S, Déry V. (2008) Revisiting Wilson and Jungner in the genomic age: a review of screening criteria over the past 40 years. *Bulletin of the World Health Organization* **86**: 317–19.

Andrew J. (1975) 'British colposcopy before the 1960s', paper presented to the 14th annual scientific meeting of the British Society of Clinical Cytology, 22–24 September 1975, University of Sussex, Brighton (unpublished, see note 68).

Anon. (1965) Clinical cytology. *British Medical Journal* **ii**: 1178.

Anon. (1966) Progress in cervical cancer testing. *British Medical Journal* **ii**: 1083.

Anon. (1968) Editorial: management of cervical carcinoma-in-situ. *Lancet* **ii**: 548–9.

Anon. (1973) Editorial: uncertainties of cervical cytology. *British Medical Journal* **ii**: 501–2.

Anon. (1985) Editorial: cervical cancer: death by incompetence. *Lancet* **326**: 363–4.

Anon. (2005) Obituary: Elizabeth Macgregor. *The Times* (21 November).

Anon. (2008) Vaccination against human papillomavirus. *Drug and Therapeutics Bulletin* **12**: 89–93.

Anttila A, Hakama M, Kotaniemi-Talonen L, Nieminen P. (2006) Alternative technologies in cervical cancer screening: a randomised evaluation trial. *BMC Public Health* **6**: 252. Freely available at http://www.biomedcentral.com/1471-2458/6/252 (visited 7 August 2009).

Anttila A, Ronco G, Clifford G, Bray F, Hakama M, Arbyn M, Weiderpass E. (2004) Cervical cancer screening programmes and policies in 18 European countries. *British Journal of Cancer* **91**: 935–41.

Attwood M E, McLaren H C, Taylor C W. (1956) The value of cytology in gynaecology. *Journal of Obstetrics and Gynaecology of the British Empire* **63**: 801–11.

Austoker J. (1994) Cancer prevention in primary care: screening for cervical cancer. *British Medical Journal* **309**: 241–8.

Ayre J E. (1949) The vaginal smear; pre-cancer cell studies using a modified technique. *American Journal of Obstetrics and Gynecology* **58**: 1205–19.

Ayre J E. (1960) Role of the halo cell in cervical cancerigenesis. A virus manifestation in premalignancy? *Obstetrics and Gynecology* **15**: 481–91.

Ayre J E, Ayre W B. (1949) Progression from pre-cancer state to early carcinoma of cervix within one year; combined cytologic and histologic study with report of case. *American Journal of Clinical Pathology* **19**: 770–8.

Babeş A. (1928) Le diagnostique du cancer du col uterin par les frottis. *La Presse Médicale* **36**: 451–4.

Babeş A. (1931). Sur le cancer superficiel du col uterin. *Gynocologie et Obstetrique* **23**: 417–33.

Barnabas R V, Laukkanen P, Koskela P, Kontula O, Lehtinen M, Garnett G P. (2006) Epidemiology of HPV 16 and cervical cancer in Finland and the potential impact of vaccination: mathematical modelling analyses. *Public Library of Science Medicine* **3**: e138, at: www.plosmedicine.org/article/info%3Adoi%2F10.1371%2Fjournal.pmed.0030138.

Barr W T, Powell D E, Raffan J B. (1970) Cellular contamination during automatic and manual staining of cytological smears. *Journal of Clinical Pathology* **23**: 604–7.

Basilico C. (1984) The mechanism of cell transformation by SV40 and polyoma virus. *Pharmacology and Therapeutics* **26**: 235–72.

Bell S, Porter M, Kitchener H, Fraser C, Fisher P, Mann E. (1995). Psychological response to cervical screening. *Preventive Medicine* **24**: 610–16.

Bentley E, Cotton S C, Cruickshank M E, Duncan I, Gray N M, Jenkins D, Little J, Neal K, Philips Z, Russell I, Seth R, Sharp L, Waugh N (The Trial of Management of Borderline and Other Low-Grade Abnormal Smears (TOMBOLA) group). (2006) Refining the management of low-grade cervical abnormalities in the UK National Health Service and defining the potential for human papillomavirus testing: a commentary on emerging evidence. *Journal of Lower Genital Tract Disease* **10**: 26–38.

Beral V. (1974) Cancer of the cervix: a sexually transmitted infection? *Lancet* **i**: 1037–40.

Beral V, Booth M. (1986) Prediction of cervical cancer incidence and mortality in England and Wales. *Lancet* **327**: 495.

Beral V (Million Women Study Collaborators). (2003) Breast cancer and hormone-replacement therapy in the Million Women Study. *Lancet* **362**: 419–27.

Beresford J M, Gervaize P A. (1986) The emotional impact of abnormal Pap smears on patients referred for colposcopy. *Colposcopy and Gynecologic Laser Surgery* **2**: 83–7.

Blanks RG, Moss S M, McGahan C E, Quinn M J, Babb P J. (2000) Effect of NHS Breast Cancer Screening Programme on mortality from breast cancer in England and Wales, 1990–89: comparison of observed with predicted mortality. *British Medical Journal* **321**: 665–9.

Bloch B, Dehaeck K, Soeters R. (eds) (1995) *Manual of Practical Gynecological Oncology*. London: Chapman and Hall Medical.

Bonnez W, Rose R C, Borkhuis C, Da Rin C, Reichman R C. (1994) Evaluation of temperature sensitivity of human papillomavirus type 11 by using the human xenograft severe combined immunodeficiency mouse model. *Journal of Clinical Microbiology* **32**: 1575–7.

Booth M, Beral V. (1989) Letter: cervical cancer deaths in young women. *Lancet* **333**: 616.

Boshart M, Gissmann L, Ikenberg H, Kleinheinz A, Scheurlen W, zur Hausen H. (1984) A new type of papillomavirus DNA, its presence in genital cancer biopsies and in cell lines derived from cervical cancer. *EMBO Journal* **3**: 1151–7.

Boyes D A, Morrison B, Knox E G, Draper G J, Miller A B. (1982) A cohort study of cervical cancer screening in British Columbia. *Clinical and Investigative Medicine* **5**: 1–29.

Bray F, Carstensen B, Møller H, Zappa M, Zakelj M P, Lawrence G, Hakama M, Weiderpass E. (2005b) Incidence trends of adenocarcinoma of the cervix in 13 European countries. *Cancer Epidemiology Biomarkers and Prevention* **14**: 2191–9.

Bray F, Loos A H, McCarron P, Weiderpass E, Arbyn M, Møller H, Hakama M, Parkin D M. (2005a) Trends in cervical squamous cell carcinoma incidence in 13 European countries: changing risk and effects of screening. *Cancer Epidemiology, Biomarkers and Prevention* **14**: 677–86.

Breslow N E, Day N E. (eds) (1987) *Statistical Methods in Cancer Research.* Vol. 2. *The design and analysis of cohort studies,* International Agency for Research on Cancer scientific publications no. 8. Lyons: IARC.

British Society for Clinical Cytology. (1983) *British Society for Clinical Cytology, 1961–83.* London: BSCC.

Bryant J, Stevens A. (1995) *Cervical Screening Interval.* Bristol: National Health Service, South and West Regional Health Authority.

Bryder L. (2008) Debates about cervical screening: an historical overview. *Journal of Epidemiology and Community Health* **62**: 284–7.

Buckley J D, Harris R W, Doll R, Vessey M P, Williams P T. (1981) Case-control study of the husbands of women with dysplasia or carcinoma of the cervix uteri. *Lancet* **318**: 1010–15.

Bulkmans N W, Berkhof J, Rozendaal L, van Kemenade FJ, Boeke AJ, Bulk S, Voorhorst F J, Verheijen R H, van Groningen K, Boon M E, Ruitinga W, van Ballegooijen M, Snijders P J, Meijer C J. (2007) Human papillomavirus DNA testing for the detection of cervical intraepithelial neoplasia grade 3 and cancer: 5-year follow-up of a randomised controlled implementation trial. *Lancet* **370**: 1764–72.

Burghardt E, Holzer E, Jordan J A. (eds) (1978) *Cervical Pathology and Colposcopy. Selected Papers from the Second World Congress of Cervical Pathology and Colposcopy.* Stuttgart: George Thieme.

Cameron D, Jones I G. (1978) Letter: sperm basic proteins in cervical carcinogenesis. *Lancet* **213**: 366.

Campion M J, Singer A, Clarkson P K, McCance D J. (1985) Increased risk of cervical neoplasia in consorts of men with penile condylomata acuminata. *Lancet* **i**: 943–6.

Campion M J, McCance D J, Cuzick J, Singer A. (1986) Progressive potential of mild cervical atypia: prospective cytological, colposcopic, and virological study. *Lancet* **ii**: 237–40.

Campion M J, Brown J R, McCance D J, Atia W, Edwards R, Cuzick J, Singer A. (1988) Psychosexual trauma of an abnormal smear. *British Journal of Obstetrics and Gynaecology* **95**: 175–81.

Campo M S, Jarrett W F H, Grindlay G J, Chandrachud L M, McGarvie G M, O'Neil B W. (1993) Prophylactic and therapeutic vaccination against a mucosal papillomavirus. *Journal of General Virology* **74**: 945–53.

Cartwright S. (1988) *The Report of the Cervical Cancer Inquiry*. Auckland, NZ: Government Printing Office.

Castle P E, Scarinci I. (2009) Should HPV vaccine be given to men? *British Medical Journal* (8 October) **339**: b4127. doi: 10.1136/bmj.b4127.

Castle P E, Lörincz A T, Scott D R, Sherman M E, Glass A G, Rush B B, Wacholder S, Burk R D, Manos M M, Schussler J E, Macomber P, Schiffman M. (2003) Comparison between prototype hybrid capture 3 and hybrid capture 2 human papillomavirus DNA assays for detection of high-grade cervical intraepithelial neoplasia and cancer. *Journal of Clinical Microbiology* **41**: 4022–30.

Chamberlain J. (1986) Reasons that some screening programmes fail to control cervical cancer. In Hakama M, Miller A B, Day N E. (eds) *Screening for Cancer of the Uterine Cervix*, IARC Scientific Publications no. 76. Lyons: IARC: 161–8.

Chan J K, Berek J S. (2007) Impact of the human papilloma vaccine on cervical cancer. *Journal of Clinical Oncology* **25**: 2975–82.

Clavel C, Masure M, Putaud I, Thomas K, Bory JP, Gabriel R, Quereux C, Birembaut P. (1998) Hybrid capture II, a new sensitive test for human papillomavirus detection. Comparison with hybrid capture I and PCR results in cervical lesions. *Journal of Clinical Pathology* **51**: 737–40.

Cochrane A L. (1972) *Effectiveness and Efficiency: Random reflections on health services*, The Rock Carling Fellowship 1971. London: Nuffield Provincial Hospitals Trust.

Cochrane A L, Holland W W. (1971) Validation of screening procedures. *British Medical Bulletin* **27**: 3–8.

Cockcroft L. (2009) Jade Goody case sparks cervical cancer test row. *Daily Telegraph* (17 February). Also at www.telegraph.co.uk/news/newstopics/celebritynews/4677821/Jade-Goody-case-sparks-cervical-cancer-test-row.html.

Colville E A, Wenban J. (1972) Letter: women returning to medicine. *British Medical Journal* **ii**: 350.

Cope J U, Hildesheim A, Schiffman M H, Manos M M, Lörincz A T, Burk R D, Glass A G, Greer C, Buckland J, Helgesen K, Scott D R, Sherman M E, Kurman R J, Liaw K L. (1997) Comparison of the hybrid capture tube test and PCR for detection of human papillomavirus DNA in cervical specimens. *Journal of Clinical Microbiology* **35**: 2262–5.

Coppleson M. (1970) The origin and nature of premalignant lesions of the cervix uteri. *International Journal of Gynecology and Obstetrics* **8**: 539–41.

Coppleson M, Reid B L. (1966) A colposcopic study of the cervix during pregnancy and the puerperium. *Journal of Obstetrics and Gynaecology of the British Commonwealth* **73**: 575–85.

Coppleson M, Reid B L. (1969) Interpretation of changes in the uterine cervix. *Lancet* **ii**: 216–17.

Coppleson M, Reid B L, Pixley E. (1967) *Preclinical Carcinoma of the Cervix Uteri: Its nature, origin and management.* Oxford; London; New York, NY: Pergamon Press.

Coppleson M, Pixley E, Reid B L. (1971) *Colposcopy: A scientific and practical approach to the cervix in health and disease.* Springfield, IL: Charles C Thomas.

Cotton S C, Sharp L, Seth R, Masson L F, Little J, Cruickshank M E, Neal K, Waugh N (TOMBOLA group). (2007) Lifestyle and socio-demographic factors associated with high-risk HPV infection in UK women. *British Journal of Cancer* **97**: 133–9.

Cotton S C, Sharp L, Little J, Duncan I, Alexander L, Cruickshank M E, Gray N M, Jenkins D, Philips Z, Robertson A, Seth R (The TOMBOLA group). (2006) Trial of management of borderline and other low-grade abnormal smears (TOMBOLA): Trial design. *Contemporary Clinical Trials* **27**: 449–71.

Crabbe J G, Egerton M E. (1961) Plea for greater use of cytological studies in early detection of cancer. *British Medical Journal* **i**: 1790–3.

Cubie H A. (1976) Failure to produce warts on human skin grafts on 'nude' mice. *British Journal of Dermatology* **94**: 659–65.

Cubie H A, Plumstead M, Zhang W, de Jesus O, Duncan L A, Stanley M A. (1998) Presence of antibodies to human papillomavirus virus-like particles (VLPs) in 11–13-year-old schoolgirls. *Journal of Medical Virology* **56**: 210–16.

Cuzick J, Sasieni P. (2001) Natural history of cervical human papillomavirus. *Lancet* **358**: 1550–1.

Cuzick J, Meijer C J, Walboomers J M. (1998a) Screening for cervical cancer. *Lancet* **351**: 1439–40.

Cuzick J, Terry G, Ho L, Hollingworth T, Anderson M. (1994) Type-specific human papillomavirus DNA in abnormal smears as a predictor of high-grade cervical intraepithelial neoplasia. *British Journal of Cancer* **69**: 167–71.

Cuzick J, Szarewski A, Terry G, Ho L, Hanby A, Maddox P, Anderson M, Kocjan G, Steele S T, Guillebaud J. (1995) Human papillomavirus testing in primary cervical screening. *Lancet* **345**: 1533–6.

Cuzick J, Holland R, Barth V, Davies R, Faupel M, Fentiman I, Frischbier H J, LaMarque J L, Merson M, Sacchini V, Vanel D, Veronesi U. (1998b) Electropotential measurements as a new diagnostic modality for breast cancer. *Lancet* **352**: 359–63.

Cuzick J, Szarewski A, Cubie H, Hulman G, Kitchener H, Luesley D, McGoogan E, Menon U, Terry G, Edwards R, Brooks C, Desai M, Gie C, Ho L, Jacobs I, Pickles C, Sasieni P. (2003) Management of women who test positive for high-risk types of human papillomavirus: the HART study. *Lancet* **362**: 1871–6.

Cuzick J, Szarewski A, Mesher D, Cadman L, Austin J, Perryman K, Ho L, Terry G, Sasieni P, Dina R, Soutter W P. (2008) Long-term follow-up of cervical abnormalities among women screened by HPV testing and cytology: results from the Hammersmith study. *International Journal of Cancer* **122**: 2294–300.

Dartmann K, Schwarz E, Gissmann L, zur Hausen H. (1986) The nucleotide sequence and genome organization of human papilloma virus type 11. *Virology* **151**: 124–30.

Day N E. (1986) The epidemiological basis for evaluating different screening programmes. In Hakama M, Miller A B, Day N E (eds) *Screening for Cancer of the Uterine Cervix*, IARC scientific publication no. 76. Lyons: International Agency for Research on Cancer: 199–209.

Department of Health. (1989) *General Practice in the National Health Service: The 1990 contract: The Government's programme for changes to GP's terms of service and remuneration system, issued by the Health Departments of Great Britain.* London: Health Departments of Great Britain.

Department of Health and Social Security, Committee on Gynaecological Cytology. (1981) *Report: Age and frequency of screening*, unpublished. Copies were available on request in 1982 from DHSS, HS1CX division, Room 1213, Hannibal House, London, SE1 6TE.

Department of Health and Social Security. (1984) *Health Services Development: Screening for cervical cancer*, HC(84)17. London: DHSS.

Department of Health and Social Security. (1986a) *Health Service Management: Cervical cancer screening*, HN(86). London: DHSS.

Department of Health and Social Security. (1986b) *Breast Cancer Screening: Report to the Health Ministers of England, Wales, Scotland and Northern Ireland by a working group chaired by Professor Sir Patrick Forrest.* London: HMSO.

Department of Health and Social Security. (1988) *Health Services Management: Cervical cancer screening*, HC(88)1. London: DHSS.

Draper G J, Cook G A. (1983) Changing patterns of cervical cancer rates. *British Medical Journal* **287**: 510–12.

Duncan I D. (1987) President's Corner. *Colposcopy and Gynecologic Laser Surgery* **3**: 3–4.

Duncan I D. (ed.) (1992) *Guidelines for Clinical Practice and Programme Management*. Oxford: NHS Cervical Screening Programme National Co-ordinating Network.

Duncan I D. (ed.) (1997) *Guidelines for Clinical Management and Programme Management*, 2nd edn, NHSCSP publication no 8. Sheffield: NHS Cervical Screening Programme.

Duncan I D. (2004) Cervical screening. *The Obstetrician and Gynaecologist* **6**: 93–7.

Dunn A E G, Ogilvie M M. (1968) Intranuclear virus particles in human genital wart tissue: observations on the ultrastructure of the epidermal layer. *Journal of Ultrastructure and Molecular Structure Research* **22**: 282–95.

Dürst M, Gissmann L, Ikenberg H, zur Hausen H. (1983) A papillomavirus DNA from a cervical carcinoma and its prevalence in cancer biopsy samples from different geographic regions. *Proceedings of the National Academy of Sciences of the USA* **80**: 3812–15.

Ebrey P B. (1996) *The Cambridge Illustrated History of China*. Cambridge: Cambridge University Press.

Einarson L. (1932) A method for progressive selective staining of Nissl and nuclear substance in nerve cells. *American Journal of Pathology* **8**: 295–305.

Evans D M, Hudson E A, Brown C L, Boddington M M, Hughes H E, Mackenzie E F. (1987) Management of women with abnormal cervical smears: supplement to terminology in gynaecological cytopathology. *Journal of Clinical Pathology* **40**: 530–1.

Evans D M, Hudson E A, Brown C L, Boddington M M, Hughes H E, Mackenzie E F, Marshall T. (1986) Terminology in gynaecological cytopathology: report of the Working Party of the British Society for Clinical Cytology. *Journal of Clinical Pathology* **39**: 933–44.

Farmery E, Gray J A M (1994). *Report of the First Five Years of the NHS Cervical Screening Programme*. Oxford: National Coordinating Network.

Franco E L, Cuzick J, Hildesheim A, de Sanjose S. (2006) Chapter 20: issues in planning cervical cancer screening in the era of HPV vaccination. *Vaccine* **24** (Suppl. 3): S171–7.

Fremont-Smith M, Graham R M. (1952) Screening for cervical cancer in internist's office by routine vaginal smears. *Journal of the American Medical Association* **150**: 587–90.

Fruin A H, Tighe J R. (1967) Tubal metaplasia of the endometrium. *Journal of Obstetrics and Gynaecology of the British Commonwealth* **74**: 93–7.

FUTURE II Study Group. (2007) Quadrivalent vaccine against human papillomavirus to prevent high-grade cervical lesions. *New England Journal of Medicine* **356**: 1915–27.

Galloway D A, Copple C D, McDougall J K. (1980) Analysis of viral DNA sequences in hamster cells transformed by herpes simplex virus type 2. *Proceedings of the National Academy of Sciences of the USA* **77**: 880–4.

Garnett G P, Kim J J, French K, Goldie S J. (2006) Chapter 21: Modelling the impact of HPV vaccines on cervical cancer and screening programmes. *Vaccine* **24** (Suppl. 3): 178–86.

Gilman M, Gilman S L, Johns J J. (2009) Human papillomavirus, abstinence and the other risks. *Lancet* **373**: 1420–1.

Gissmann L, zur Hausen H. (1976) Human papillomaviruses: physical mapping and genetic heterogeneity. *Proceedings of the National Academy of Sciences of the USA* **73**: 1310–13.

Gissmann L, zur Hausen H. (1980) Partial characterization of viral DNA from human genital warts (condylomata acuminata). *International Journal of Cancer* **25**: 605–9.

Gissmann L, Diehl V, Schultz-Coulon H J, zur Hausen H. (1982) Molecular cloning and characterization of human papilloma virus DNA derived from a laryngeal papilloma. *Journal of Virology* **44**: 393–400.

Glucksmann A, Way S, Cherry C P. (1964) The ten-year results of individualized treatment of carcinoma of the cervix based on the analysis of serial biopsies. *Journal of Obstetrics and Gynaecology of the British Commonwealth* **71**: 198–201.

Goldie S J, Kim J J, Wright T C. (2004) Cost-effectiveness of human papillomavirus DNA testing for cervical cancer screening in women aged 30 years or more. *Obstetrics and Gynecology* **103**: 619–31.

Goldie S J, Freedberg K A, Weinstein M C, Wright T C, Kuntz K M. (2001) Cost effectiveness of human papillomavirus testing to augment cervical cancer screening in women infected with the human immunodeficiency virus. *American Journal of Medicine* **111**: 140–9.

Goldman J M, Epstein M A. (eds) (1986) *Vaccine Intervention Against Virus-induced Tumours*, Leukaemia and lymphoma research series no. 3. Basingstoke: Macmillan.

Graham R M. (1963) *The Cytologic Diagnosis of Cancer*, 2nd edn. Philadelphia, PA: Saunders.

Gray J A M. (1990) *General Principles of Quality Assurance in Breast Cancer Screening*. Oxford: National Health Service Breast Screening Programme.

Gray J A M. (1997) Evidence-based, locally owned, patient-centred guideline development. *British Journal of Surgery* **84**: 1636–7.

Gray J A M. (2004) Evidence-based policy making. *British Medical Journal* **329**: 988–9.

Gray N M, Sharp L, Cotton S C, Avis M, Philips Z, Russell I, Walker L G, Whynes D, Little J (TOMBOLA group). (2005) Developing a questionnaire to measure the psychosocial impact of an abnormal cervical smear result and its subsequent management: the TOMBOLA (Trial of Management of Borderline and Other Low-grade Abnormal Smears) trial. *Quality of Life Research* **14**: 1553–62.

Gray N M, Sharp L, Cotton S C, Masson L F, Little J, Walker L G, Avis M, Philips Z, Russell I, Whynes D, Cruickshank M, Woolley C M (TOMBOLA group). (2006) Psychological effects of a low-grade abnormal cervical smear test result: anxiety and associated factors. *British Journal of Cancer* **94**: 1253–62.

Gray W, McKee G T. (2003) *Diagnostic Cytopathology*, 2nd edn. Edinburgh: Churchill Livingstone.

Green A, Beral V, Moser K. (1988) Mortality in women in relation to their childbearing history. *British Medical Journal* **297**: 391–5.

Griffiths M. (1991) Nuns, virgins, and spinsters: Rigoni-Stern and cervical cancer revisited. *British Journal of Obstetrics and Gynaecology* **98**: 797–802.

Guthrie D, Ross W M, Latner A L, Turner G A, Way S. (1981) Effective treatment of a patient with an advanced carcinoma of the cervix with a combination of bromocriptine and aprotinin. *British Journal of Clinical Practice* **35**: 330–2.

Hakama M. (1982) Trends in the incidence of cervical cancer in the Nordic countries, in Magnus K. (ed.) *Trends in Cancer Incidence: Causes and practical implications*, Proceedings of a symposium held in Oslo, Norway, 6–7 August 1980. Washington, DC: Hemisphere Publishing Corporation for the International Union Against Cancer and the Norwegian Cancer Society: 279–92.

Hakama M. (1990) A screening programme that worked: discussion paper. *Journal of the Royal Society of Medicine* **83**: 322–4.

Hakama M, Miller A B, Day N E. (eds) (1986) *Screening for Cancer of the Uterine Cervix*. Lyons: IARC Scientific Publications.

zur Hausen H. (1975) Oncogenic herpes viruses. *Biochimica et Biophysica Acta* **417**: 25–53.

zur Hausen H. (1976) Condylomata acuminata and human genital cancer. *Cancer Research* **36**: 794.

zur Hausen H. (1987) Papillomaviruses in human cancer. *Applied Pathology* **5**: 19–24.

zur Hausen H. (2006) *Infections Causing Human Cancer*. Weinheim: Wiley-VCH.

zur Hausen H, Meinhof W, Scheiber W, Bornkamm G W. (1974) Attempts to detect virus-specific DNA in human tumors. I. Nucleic acid hybridizations with complementary RNA of human wart virus. *International Journal of Cancer* **13**: 650–6.

Havelock C M, Webb J, Queenborough J. (1988) Preliminary results of a district call scheme for cervical screening organised in general practice. *British Medical Journal* **297**: 1384–6.

Herbert A. (ed.) (1995) Achievable standards benchmarks for reporting, criteria for evaluating cervical cytopathology, NHSCSP publication no. 1. Sheffield: NHS Cervical Screening Programme.

Herbert A. (2000) Cervical screening in England and Wales: its effect has been underestimated. *Cytopathology* **11**: 471–9.

Herbert A. (2009) (Janet) Elizabeth Macgregor (1920–2005). *Oxford Dictionary of National Biography*, online edn. Oxford: Oxford University Press. Also available at www.oxforddnb.com/view/article/96184 (visited 16 September 2009).

Herbert A, Anshu, Gregory M, Gupta S S, Singh N. (2009) Invasive cervical cancer audit: a relative increase in interval cancers while coverage increased and incidence declined. *BJOG* **116**: 845–53.

Hill G B, Adelstein A M. (1967) Cohort mortality from carcinoma of the cervix. *Lancet* **ii**: 605–6.

Hinselmann H. (1925) Verbesserung der Inspektionsmöglichkeiten von Vulva, Vagina und Portio. *Münchener Medizinische Wochenschrift* **72**: 1733-40.

Hinsey J C. (1962) George Nicholas Papanicolaou, 13 May 1883–19 February 1962. *Acta Cytologica* **6**: 483–6.

House of Commons, Committee of Public Accounts. (1992) *Cervical and Breast Screening in England*, HoC 58, Session 1992/3. London: HMSO.

Howe A, Owen-Smith V, Richardson J. (2002) The impact of a television soap opera on the NHS Cervical Screening Programme in the North West of England. *Journal of Public Health Medicine* **24**: 299–304.

Howe A, Owen-Smith V, Richardson J. (2003) Letter: media influence on suicide: television programme makers have an ethical responsibility. *British Medical Journal* **326**: 498.

Husain O A N. (1972) St Stephen's Hospital group. *British Medical Journal* **iii**: 769.

Husain O A N. (1988) S A Way. *British Medical Journal* **297**: 915.

Husain O A N, Butler E B. (1999) Training in cervical cytology. *Cytopathology* **10**: 420.

Husain O A N, Mackenzie E F D, Walter D. (1970) The Quantimet: an image analyzing computer. *Acta Cytologica* **14**: 160.

Imperial Cancer Research Fund, Coordinating Committee on Cervical Screening. (1984) Organization of a programme for cervical cancer screening. *British Medical Journal* **289**: 894–5.

Imperial Cancer Research Fund, Coordinating Committee on Cervical Screening. (1986) The management of a cervical screening programme: a statement (October 1985). *Community Medicine* **8**: 179–84.

International Agency for Research on Cancer (IARC) Working Group on evaluation of cervical cancer screening programmes. (1986) Screening for squamous cervical cancer: duration of low risk after negative results of cervical cytology and its implication for screening policies. *British Medical Journal* **293**: 659–64.

JKR. (1988) Obituary: S A Way. *British Medical Journal* **297**: 550.

Jarrett W F H. (1978) Transformation of warts to malignancy in alimentary carcinoma in cattle. *Bulletin du Cancer* **65**: 191–4.

Jarrett W F H, Murphy J, O'Neil B W, Laird H M. (1978b) Virus-induced papillomas of the alimentary tract of cattle. *International Journal of Cancer* **22**: 323–8.

Jarrett W F H, McNeil P E, Grimshaw W T, Selman I E, McIntyre W I. (1978a) High incidence area of cattle cancer with a possible interaction between an environmental carcinogen and a papilloma virus. *Nature* **274**: 215–17.

Jenkins D. (2006) Public health issues related to HPV vaccination. In Monsonego J. (ed.) *Emerging Issues on HPV Infections: From science to practice.* Basel; London: Karger: 253–65.

Jit M, Choi Y H, Edmunds W J. (2008) Economic evaluation of human papillomavirus vaccination in the United Kingdom. *British Medical Journal* **337**: a769.

Johnson A M, Wadsworth J, Wellings K, Bradshaw S, Field J. (1992) Sexual lifestyles and HIV risk. *Nature* **360**: 410–12.

Johnson A M, Wadsworth J, Wellings K, Field J, with Sally Bradshaw. (1994) *Sexual Attitudes and Lifestyles.* Oxford: Blackwell Scientific Publications.

Johnson J, Patnick J. (eds) (2000) *Achievable Standards, Benchmarks for Reporting, Criteria for Evaluating Cervical Cytopathology*, 2nd edn, including revised performance indicators, NHSCSP publication no. 1. Sheffield: NHS Cervical Screening Programme.

Jones R W. (2009) A medical journal editor's role in exposing an unethical research study. *Obstetrics and Gynecology* **113**: 161–5.

Jordan J A. (1975) The present situation of colposcopy: GB. Paper presented at the 2nd World Congress of Cervical Pathology and Colposcopy, Graz, Austria. Unpublished; copy to be deposited with records of meeting. See note 68.

Jordan J A, Sharp F, Singer A. (eds). (1982). *Pre-Clinical Neoplasia of the Cervix:* Proceedings of the ninth study group of the Royal College of Obstetricians and Gynaecologists, October 1981. London: RCOG.

Kassirer E. (1980) Impact of the Walton report on cervical cancer screening programs in Canada. *Canadian Medical Association Journal* **122**: 417–23.

Kinlen L J, Spriggs A I. (1978) Women with positive cervical smears but without surgical intervention. A follow-up study. *Lancet* **ii**: 463–5.

Kitchener H C. (1988) Commentary: does HPV cause cervical cancer? *British Journal of Obstetrics and Gynaecology* **95**: 1089–91.

Kitchener H C, Neilson L, Burnett R A, Young L, Macnab J C M. (1991) Prospective serial study of viral change in the cervix and correlation with human papillomavirus genome status. *British Journal of Obstetrics and Gynaecology* **98**: 1042–8.

Kmietowicz Z. (2008) Opportunity was missed in choice of cervical cancer vaccine, health campaigners say. *British Medical Journal* **336**: 1456–7.

Knox E G. (1966) Cervical cytology: a scrutiny of the evidence. In McLachlan G. (ed.) *Problems and Progress in Medical Care: Essays on current research*, 2nd series. London: Oxford University Press: 277–307.

Kolstad P. (1970) Diagnosis and management of precancerous lesions of the cervix uteri. *International Journal of Gynecology and Obstetrics* **8**: 551–60.

Koss L G. (1961) *Diagnostic Cytology and its Histopathologic Bases*, 1st edn in association with Grace R Durfee. London: Pitman Medical Publishing Co.; Philadelphia, PA: J B Lippincott Co.

Koss L G. (1975) *Tumors of the Urinary Bladder*, atlas of tumor pathology series, fasc.11. ser. 2. Washington, DC: Armed Forces Institute of Pathology.

Koss L G. (1987) Cytologic and histologic manifestations of human papillomavirus infection of the female genital tract and their clinical significance. *Cancer* **60** (Suppl.): 1942–50.

Koss L G. (1989) Cytologic diagnosis of human cancer: a Citation Classic commentary *On Diagnostic Cytology and its Histopathologic Bases* by L G Koss (1961). *Current Contents: Life Sciences* **32**: 15

Koss L G. (2007) Of tissues, cells, and molecules: reminiscences of an old pathologist. *Human Pathology* **38**: 1447–53.

Koss L G, Durfee G R. (1956) Unusual patterns of squamous epithelium of the uterine cervix: cytologic and pathologic study of koilocytotic atypia. *Annals of the New York Academy of Sciences* **63**: 1245–61.

Koss L G, Melamed M R. (eds) (2006) *Koss' Diagnostic Cytology and its Histopathologic Bases*, 5th edn, 2 vols. Philadelphia, PA: Lippincott Williams and Wilkins.

Koss L G, Stewart F, Foote F W, Jordan M J, Bader G M, Day E. (1963) Some histological aspects of behavior of epidermoid carcinoma *in situ* (CIS) and related lesions of the uterine cervix. A long-term prospective study. *Cancer* **16**: 1160–211.

Kotaniemi-Talonen L, Malila N, Nieminen P, Anttila A, Tarkkanen J, Laurila P, Hakama M. (2008a) Test positivity cut-off level of a high risk human papillomavirus test could be increased in routine cervical cancer screening. *International Journal of Cancer* **123**: 2902–6.

Kotaniemi-Talonen L, Anttila A, Malila N, Tarkkanen J, Laurila P, Hakama M, Nieminen P. (2008b) Screening with a primary human papillomavirus test does not increase detection of cervical cancer and intraepithelial neoplasia 3. *European Journal of Cancer* **44**: 565–71.

Lane D P, Crawford L V. (1979) T antigen is bound to a host protein in SV40-transformed cells. *Nature* **278**: 261–3.

Langley F A, Crompton A C. (1973) *Epithelial Abnormalities of the Cervix Uteri*, recent results in cancer research series no. 40. London: Heinemann Medical.

Laverty C R, Russell P, Hills E, Booth N. (1978) The significance of non-condyloma wart virus infection of the cervical transformation zone. A review with discussion of two illustrative cases. *Acta Cytologica* **22**: 195–201.

Law M R, Morris J K, Wald N J. (1999) The importance of age in screening for cancer. *Journal of Medical Screening* **6**: 16–20.

Lawler S D. (1981) Conception and development of the fetal tissue bank. *Journal of Clinical Pathology* **34**: 240–8.

Legood R, Gray A, Wolstenholme J, Moss S. (2006) Lifetime effects, costs, and cost effectiveness of testing for human papillomavirus to manage low grade cytological abnormalities: results of the NHS pilot studies. *British Medical Journal* **332**: 79–85.

Levine A J. (1976) SV40 and adenovirus early functions involved in DNA replication and transformation. *Biochim Biophys Acta* **458**: 213–41.

Levine A J. (1990) Tumor suppressor genes. *Bioessays* **12**: 60–6.

Lörincz A T, Temple G F, Patterson J A, Jenson A B, Kurman R J, Lancaster W D. (1986) Correlation of cellular atypia and human papillomavirus deoxyribonucleic acid sequences in exfoliated cells of the uterine cervix. *Obstetrics and Gynaecology* **68**: 508–12.

Lucasson J-F, McNab D, Collins T C, Mattingley J R, Keen J N, MacLean A B, Macnab J C M. (1994) HSV-2 increases the mitochondrial aspartate amino transaminase characteristic of tumor cells. *Virology* **205**: 393–405.

Luesley D. (ed.) (1996) *Standards and Quality in Colposcopy*, NHSCSP publication no. 2. Sheffield: NHS Cervical Screening Programme.

Luesley D, Leeson S. (eds) (2004) *Colposcopy and Programme Management*, NHSCSP publication no. 20. Sheffield: NHS Cervical Screening Programme.

Macgregor J E. (1981) *Taking Uterine Cervical Smears*, BSCC publication. Aberdeen: Aberdeen University Press.

Macgregor J E, Baird D. (1963) Detection of cervical carcinoma in the general population. *British Medical Journal* **i**: 1631–6.

Macgregor J E, Teper S. (1974) Letter: screening for cervical cancer. *Lancet* **303**: 1221.

Macgregor J E, Fraser M E, Mann E M F. (1971) Improved prognosis of cervical cancer due to comprehensive screening. *Lancet* **297**: 74–6.

Macgregor J E, Campbell M K, Mann E M, Swanson K Y. (1994) Screening for cervical intraepithelial neoplasia in north east Scotland shows fall in incidence and mortality from invasive cancer with concomitant rise in pre-invasive disease. *British Medical Journal* **308**: 1407–11.

Macgregor J E, Moss S M, Parkin D M, Day N E. (1985) A case-control study of cervical cancer screening in north east Scotland. *British Medical Journal* **290**: 1543–6.

Macgregor J E, Moss S, Parkin D M. (1986) Cervical cancer screening in North East Scotland, in Hakama M, Miller A B, Day N E. (eds) *Screening for Cancer of the Uterine Cervix.* Lyons: IARC Scientific Publications: 25–36.

Macnab J C M, Walkinshaw S A, Cordiner J W, Clements J B. (1986) Human papillomavirus in clinically and histologically normal tissue of patients with genital cancer. *New England Journal of Medicine* **315**: 1052–8.

Marteau T M, Walker P, Giles J, Smail M. (1990) Anxieties in women undergoing colposcopy. *British Journal of Obstetrics and Gynaecology* **97**: 859–61.

Matlashewski G. (1989) The cell biology of human papillomavirus transformed cells. *Anticancer Research* **9**: 1447–56.

Mayrand M H, Duarte-Franco E, Rodrigues I, Walter S D, Hanley J, Ferenczy A, Ratnam S, Coutlée F, Franco E L; Canadian Cervical Cancer Screening Trial Study Group. (2007) Human papillomavirus DNA versus Papanicolaou screening tests for cervical cancer. *New England Journal of Medicine* **357**: 1579–88.

McCaffery K, Waller J, Forrest S, Cadman L, Szarewski A, Wardle J. (2004) Testing positive for human papillomavirus in routine cervical screening: examination of the psychosocial impact. *BJOG* **111**: 1437–43.

McCance D J, Campion M J, Clarkson P K, Chesters P M, Jenkins D, Singer A. (1985) Prevalence of human papillomavirus type 16 DNA sequences in cervical intraepithelial neoplasia and invasive carcinoma of the cervix. *British Journal of Obstetrics and Gynaecology* **92**: 1101–5.

McCredie M R, Sharples K J, Paul C, Baranyai J, Medley G, Jones R W, Skegg D C. (2008) Natural history of cervical neoplasia and risk of invasive cancer in women with cervical intraepithelial neoplasia 3: a retrospective cohort study. *Lancet Oncology* **9**: 425–34.

McGahan C E, Blanks R G, Moss S M. (2001) Reasons for variation in coverage in the NHS cervical screening programme. *Cytopathology* **12**: 354–66.

McLachlan G. (ed.) *Problems and Progress in Medical Care: Essays on current research*, 2nd series. London: Oxford University Press.

McLaren H C, Taylor C W, Attwood M E. (1958) Cytological diagnosis in gynaecological practice. *Lancet* **i**: 398–400.

McNeil C. (2006) Who invested in the VLP cervical cancer vaccines? *Journal of the National Cancer Institute* **98**: 433.

Mant D, Vessey M, Loudon N. (1988) Social class differences in sexual behaviour and cervical cancer. *Community Medicine* **10**: 52–6.

Marais D, Rose R C, Williamson A-L. (1997) A study of the age distribution of antibodies to human papillomavirus in children, women with cervical intraepithelial neoplasia and blood donors from South Africa. *Journal of Medical Virology* **31**: 126–31.

Meisels A, Fortin R. (1976) Condylomatus lesions of the cervix and vagina. I. Cytologic patterns. *Acta Cytologica* **20**: 505–9.

Meisels A, Fortin R, Roy M. (1977) Condylomatous lesions of the cervix. II. Cytologic, colposcopic and histopathologic study. *Acta Cytologica* **21**: 379–90.

Melchers W J, Claas H C, Quint W G. (1991) Use of the polymerase chain reaction to study the relationship between human papillomavirus infections and cervical cancer. *European Journal of Clinical Microbiology and Infectious Diseases* **10**: 714–27.

Michalas S P. (2000) The Pap test: George N Papanicolaou (1883–1962). A screening test for the prevention of cancer of uterine cervix. *European Journal of Obstetrics and Gynecology and Reproductive Biology* **90**: 135–8.

Miller A B, Lindsay J, Hill G B. (1976) Mortality from cancer of the uterus in Canada and its relationship to screening for cancer of the cervix. *International Journal of Cancer* **17**: 602–12.

Ministry of Health. (1964) *Special Training Courses in Extoliative Cytology*, HM(64)70, September. London: HMSO.

Ministry of Health. (1966) *Population Screening for Cancer of the Cervix*, HM(66)76. London: HMSO.

Monsonego J. (ed.) (2006) *Emerging Issues on HPV Infections: From science to practice*. Basel; London: Karger.

Montaigne M de. (1580) *Essais*, bk 3, ch 12. In Rat M (ed.) (1996) *Oxford Dictionary of Quotations*, rev. 4th edn. Oxford: Oxford University Press: 481.

Moore R A, Walcott S, White K L, Anderson D M, Jain S, Lloyd A, Topley P, Thomsen L, Gough G W, Stanley M A. (2003) Therapeutic immunisation with COPV early genes by epithelial DNA delivery. *Virology* **314**: 630–5.

Moss S M, Gray A, Legood R, Henstock E. (2002) *Evaluation of HPV/LBC Cervical Screening Pilot Studies: First report to the Department of Health on evaluation of LBC*, revised January 2003. Freely available at: www.cancerscreening.nhs.uk/cervical/lbc-pilot-evaluation.pdf (visited 7 August 2009).

Moss S, Gray A, Legood R, Vessey M, Patnick J, Kitchener H (Liquid-based Cytology/Human Papillomavirus Cervical Pilot Studies Group). (2006) Effect of testing for human papillomavirus as a triage during screening for cervical cancer: observational before and after study. *British Medical Journal* **332**: 83–5.

Mould T A, Singer A, Gallivan S. (2000) Quantitative detection of oncogenic HPV DNA using hybrid capture to triage borderline and mildly dyskaryotic Papanicolaou smears. *European Journal of Gynaecological Oncology* **21**: 245–8.

Münger K, Baldwin A, Edwards K M, Hayakawa H, Nguyen C L, Owens M, Grace M, Huh K. (2004) Mechanisms of human papillomavirus-induced oncogenesis. *Journal of Virology* **78**: 11451–60.

National Audit Office. (1992) *Cervical and Breast Screening in England: Report by the Comptroller and Auditor General*, Session 1991/2, HC-236. London: HMSO.

National Audit Office. (1998) *The Performance of the NHS Cervical Screening Programme in England: Report by the Comptroller and Auditor General*, Session 1997/8, HC-678. London: The Stationery Office.

National Audit Office. (2009) *Department of Health: Young people's sexual health: the National Chlamydia Screening Programme, Report by the Comptroller and Auditor General,* Session 2008–09, HC-963. London: HMSO.

National Health Service Breast Screening Programme. (1991) *Breast cancer screening. (1991) Evidence and Experience since the Forrest Report.* Sheffield: NHSBSP-Trent RHA.

National Health Service Cervical Screening Programme (NHSCSP). (1996) *Quality Assurance Guidelines for the Cervical Screening Programme.* Sheffield: NHSCSP.

National Health Service Cervical Screening Programme. (2003) *Celebrating 15 Years of Achievement: Annual Review 2003.* Sheffield: NHSCSP.

National Institute for Clinical Excellence. (2003) *Guidance on the Use of Liquid-Based Cytology for Cervical Screening,* technology appraisal 69. London: NICE.

Naucler P, Ryd W, Törnberg S, Strand A, Wadell G, Elfgren K, Rådberg T, Strander B, Johansson B, Forslund O, Hansson B G, Rylander E, Dillner J. (2007) Human papillomavirus and Papanicolaou tests to screen for cervical cancer. *New England Journal of Medicine* **357**: 1589–97.

Nieminen P, Soares V R, Aho M, Vesterinen E, Savia E, Vaheri A, Paavonen J. (1991) Cervical human papillomavirus deoxyribonucleic acid and cytologic evaluations in gynecologic outpatients. *American Journal of Obstetrics and Gynecology* **164**: 1265–9.

O'Dowd A. (2009) Teenager who died after having HPV vaccine had a malignant chest tumour. *British Medical Journal* **339**: b4032 .

O'Dowd M J, Philipp E E. (1994) *The History of Obstetrics and Gynaecology.* Carnforth: Parthenon Publishing Group Ltd.

Office for National Statistics (ONS). (1999–2006) *Cancer Registration Statistics, England,* annual, online edition at: www.statistics.gov.uk/StatBase/Product.asp?vlnk=7720 (visited 8 December 2009).

Offord E A, Leake R E, Macnab J C M. (1989) Stimulation of estrogen receptor mRNA levels in MCF-7 cells by herpes simplex virus infection. *Journal of Virology* **63**: 2388–91.

Oriel J D, Almeida J D. (1970) Demonstration of virus particles in human genital warts. *British Journal of Venereal Diseases* **46**: 37–42.

Papanicolaou G N. (1928) New cancer diagnosis. *Proceedings of the Third Race Betterment Conference.* Battle Creek, MI: Race Betterment Foundation: 528–30.

Papanicolaou G N. (1954) *Atlas of Exfoliative Cytology.* Cambridge, MA: Harvard University Press; Oxford University Press for the Commonwealth Fund.

Papanicolaou G N, Traut H F. (1941) The diagnostic value of vaginal smears in carcinoma of the uterus. *American Journal of Obstetrics and Gynecology* **42**: 193–206.

Papanicolaou G N, Traut H F. (1943) *Diagnosis of Uterine Cancer by the Vaginal Smear.* New York, NY: Commonwealth Fund.

Park M, Kitchener H C, Macnab J C M. (1983) Detection of herpes simplex virus type-2 DNA restriction fragments in human cervical carcinoma tissue. *EMBO Journal* **2**: 1029–34.

Park M, Lonsdale D M, Timbury M C, Subak-Sharpe J H, Macnab J C M. (1980) Genetic retrieval of viral genome sequences from herpes simplex virus transformed cells. *Nature* **285**: 412–15.

Patnick J. (ed.) (2006) *Audit of Invasive Cervical Cancers*, NHSCSP Publication no. 28. Sheffield: NHS Cancer Screening Programmes. Freely available at: www.cancerscreening.nhs.uk/cervical/publications/nhscsp28.html (visited 27 July 2009).

Patnick J. (ed.) (2008a) *Annual Review 2007.* Sheffield: NHS CSP and freely available at www.cancerscreening.nhs.uk/cervical/publications/cervical-annual-review-2007.pdf (visited 29 April 2009)

Patnick J. (ed.) (2008b) *Celebrating 20 Years of Screening: NHS Cancer Screening Programmes.* Sheffield: NHSCSP.

Patten S F Jr. (1969) Diagnostic cytology of the uterine cervix. *Monographs in Clinical Cytology* **3**: 1–209.

Peto J, Gilham C, Fletcher O, Matthews F E. (2004a) The cervical cancer epidemic that screening has prevented in the UK. *Lancet* **364**: 249–56.

Peto J, Gilham C, Deacon J, Taylor C, Evans C, Binns W, Haywood M, Elanko N, Coleman D, Yule R, Desai M. (2004b) Cervical HPV infection and neoplasia in a large population-based prospective study: the Manchester cohort. *British Journal of Cancer* **91**: 942–53.

Peto R, zur Hausen H. (eds) (1986) *Viral Etiology of Cervical Cancer*: Based on a conference held 14–17 April 1985 at the Banbury Center of Cold Spring Harbor Laboratory. Cold Spring Harbor, Long Island, NY: Cold Spring Harbor Laboratory.

Peyton C L, Schiffman M, Lörincz A T, Hunt W C, Mielzynska I, Bratti C, Eaton S, Hildesheim A, Morera L A, Rodriguez A C, Herrero R, Sherman M E, Wheeler C M. (1998) Comparison of PCR- and hybrid capture-based human papillomavirus detection systems using multiple cervical specimen collection strategies. *Journal of Clinical Microbiology* **36**: 3248–54.

Pike C, Chamberlain J. (1992) *Guidelines on Failsafe Actions.* Oxford: NHS National Coordinating Network.

Pontén J, Adami H O, Bergström R, Dillner J, Friberg L G, Gustafsson L, Miller A B, Parkin D M, Sparén P, Trichopoulos D. (1995) Strategies for global control of cervical cancer. *International Journal of Cancer* **60**: 1–26. Comment in: *International Journal of Cancer* (1995) **63**: 315–16.

Poulsen R S, Oliver L H, Cahn R L, Louis C, Toussaint G. (1977) High resolution analysis of cervical cells: a progress report. *Journal of Histochemistry and Cytochemistry* **25**: 689–95.

Prunieras M. (ed.) (1976) *Biomedical Aspects of Human Wart Virus Infection,* proceedings of a Fondation Mérieux seminar held in Lyons 15–16 December 1975. Lyons: Fondation Mérieux.

Purola E, Savia E. (1977) Cytology of gynecologic condyloma acuminatum. *Acta Cytologica* **21**: 26–31.

Quinn M, Babb P, Jones J, Allen E on behalf of the UK Association of Cancer Registries. (1999) Effect of screening on incidence of and mortality from cancer of cervix in England: evaluation based on routinely collected statistics. *British Medical Journal* **318**: 904–8.

Raffle A E, Alden B, Quinn M, Babb PJ, Brett M T. (2003) Outcomes of screening to prevent cancer: analysis of cumulative incidence of cervical abnormality and modelling of cases and deaths prevented. *British Medical Journal* **326**: 901.

Rawls W E, Tompkins W A, Figueroa M E, Melnick J L. (1968) Herpesvirus type 2: association with carcinoma of the cervix. *Science* **161**: 1255–6.

Reagan J W, Patten S F Jr. (1962) Dysplasia: a basic reaction to injury in the uterine cervix. *Annals of the New York Academy of Sciences* **97**: 662–82.

Reid B L. (1964) The behaviour of human sperm toward cultured fragments of human cervix uteri. *Lancet* **283**: 21–3.

Reid B L, Singer A, Coppleson M. (1967) The process of cervical regeneration after electrocauterization. I. Histological and colposcopic study. *Australian and New Zealand Journal of Obstetrics and Gynaecology* **7**: 125–35.

Reid B L, French P W, Hagan B E, Coppleson M. (1978b) Letter: sperm basic proteins and cervical carcinogenesis. *Lancet* **312**: 788–9.

Reid B L, French P W, Singer A, Hagan B E, Coppleson M. (1978a) Sperm basic proteins in cervical carcinogenesis: Correlation with socioeconomic class. *Lancet* **312**: 60–2.

Rice P S, Cason J, Best J M, Banatvala J E. (1999) High risk genital papillomavirus infections are spread vertically. *Reviews in Medical Virology* **9**: 15–21.

Richardson J, Owen-Smith V, Howe A. (2002) The effect of 'Alma's' death on women attending for a cervical smear: a questionnaire survey. *Journal of Public Health Medicine* **24**: 305–6.

Richart R M. (1964) The correlation of Schiller-positive areas on the exposed portion of the cervix with intraepithelial neoplasia. *American Journal of Obstetrics and Gynecology* **90**: 696–701.

Richmond C. (2005) Janet Elizabeth Macgregor: pioneer of cervical screening. *British Medical Journal* **331**: 1410.

Riggott J M. (ed.) *The Early Diagnosis of Cancer of the Cervix*: A symposium held at the University of Hull on the 20 March 1970 as part of the 11th Annual General Meeting of the British Association for Cancer Research. Hull: University of Hull.

Rigoni-Stern D A. (1842) Fatti statistici relativi alle malattie cancerose che servirono di base alle poche cose dette dal dott. *Giornale per servire ai progressi della patologia e della terapeutica* **2**: 507–17.

Rigoni-Stern D A. (1988) Statistical facts about cancers on which Dr Rigoni-Stern based his contribution to the surgeons' subgroup of the IV Congress of the Italian Scientists on 23 September 1842 [translation from the Italian]. *Statistics in Medicine* **6**: 881–4.

Rob L. (2007) Cervical cancer screening in the Czech Republic. *Collegium Antropologicum* **31** (Suppl. 2): 27–9.

Robertson J H, Woodend B. (1993) Negative cytology preceding cervical cancer: causes and prevention. *Journal of Clinical Pathology* **46**: 700–2.

Rogstad K E. (2002) The psychological impact of abnormal cytology and colposcopy. *BJOG* **109**: 364–8.

Ronco G, Segnan N, Giorgi-Rossi P, Zappa M, Casadei G P, Carozzi F, Dalla Palma P, Del Mistro A, Folicaldi S, Gillio-Tos A, Nardo G, Naldoni C, Schincaglia P, Zorzi M, Confortini M, Cuzick J; J (New Technologies for Cervical Cancer Working Group). (2006) Human papillomavirus testing and liquid-based cytology: results at recruitment from the new technologies for cervical cancer randomized controlled trial. *Journal of the National Cancer Institute* **98**: 765–74.

Ronco G, Giorgi-Rossi P, Carozzi F, Confortini M, Dalla Palma P, Del Mistro A, Gillio-Tos A, Minucci D, Naldoni C, Rizzolo R, Schincaglia P, Volante R, Zappa M, Zorzi M, Cuzick J, Segnan N (New Technologies for Cervical Cancer Screening Working Group). (2008) Results at recruitment from a randomized controlled trial comparing human papillomavirus testing alone with conventional cytology as the primary cervical cancer screening test. *Journal of the National Cancer Institute* **100**: 492–501.

Rose R C, Reichman R C, Bonnez W. (1994a) Human papillomavirus (HPV) type 11 recombinant virus-like particles induce the formation of neutralizing antibodies and detect HPV-specific antibodies in human sera. *Journal of General Virology* **75**: 2075–9.

Rose R C, Bonnez W, Da Rin C, McCance D J, Reichman R C. (1994b) Serological differentiation of human papillomavirus types 11, 16 and 18 using recombinant virus-like particles. *Journal of General Virology* **75**: 2445–9.

Rotkin I D. (1962) Relation of adolescent coitus to cervical cancer risk. *Journal of the American Medical Association* **179**: 486–91.

Rotkin I D. (1967) Epidemiology of cancer of the cervix. 3. Sexual characteristics of a cervical cancer population. *American Journal of Public Health and the Nation's Health* **57**: 815–29.

Rotkin I D. (1973) A comparison review of key epidemiological studies in cervical cancer related to current searches for transmissible agents. *Cancer Research* **33**: 1353–67.

Royal College of Obstetricians and Gynaecologists, Royal College of Pathologists, Royal College of General Practitioners and Faculty of Community Medicine, Intercollegiate Working Party. (1987) *Report on Cervical Cytology Screening*. London: Progress Press for the Royal College of Obstetricians and Gynaecologists.

Royal College of Pathologists. (2008) *Evaluation of Clinical Events (ECE): Guidance for assessors and trainees in histopathology*. London: Royal College of Pathologists Assessment Department. Freely available at: www.rcpath.org/resources/pdf/histopathology_ece_guidance.pdf (visited 5 August 2009).

Royal College of Pathologists , British Society for Clinical Cytology and NHS Cervical Screening Programme. (1995) Achievable standards benchmarks for reporting, criteria for evaluating cervical cytopathology. *Cytopathology* **6** (Suppl. 2): 7–32.

Rue R. (1967) Employment of married women doctors in hospitals in the Oxford region. *Lancet* **i**: 1267–8.

Sagiroglu N. (1963) Progression and regression studies of precancer (anaplastic or dysplastic) cells and the halo test. *American Journal of Obstetrics and Gynecology* **85**: 454–69.

Sargent A, Bailey A, Almonte M, Turner A, Thomson C, Peto J, Desai M, Mather J, Moss S, Roberts C, Kitchener H C (ARTISTIC Study Group). (2008) Prevalence of type-specific HPV infection by age and grade of cervical cytology: data from the ARTISTIC trial. *British Journal of Cancer* **98**: 1704–9.

Sasieni P, Adams J. (1999) Effect of screening on cervical cancer mortality in England and Wales: analysis of trends with an age period cohort model. *British Medical Journal* **318**: 1244–5.

Sasieni P D, Adams J, Cuzick J. (2003) Benefit of cervical screening at different ages: evidence from the UK audit of screening histories. *British Journal of Cancer* **89**: 88–93.

Sasieni P D, Cuzick J, Lynch-Farmery E and the NCN Working Group. (1996) Estimating the efficacy of screening by auditing smear histories of women with and without cervical cancer. *British Journal of Cancer* **73**: 1001–5.

Savard M. (2006) Bridging the communication gap between practitioners and their patients: role of HPV and advances in cervical cancer prevention, in Monsonego J. (ed.) *Emerging Issues in HPV Infections: From science to practice.* Basel: Karger: 44–53.

Sawin C T. (2002) George N Papanicolaou and the 'Pap' test. *Endocrinologist* **12**: 267–72.

Schauenstein W. (1908) Histologische Untersuchungen uber atypisches Plattenepithel an der Portio und an der Innenflache der Cervix uteri. *Archiv für Gynäkologie* **85**: 576–616.

Schiffman M, Castle P E. (2006) Editorial: when to test women for human papillomavirus: cervical screening using HPV testing shows great promise but warrants caution. *British Medical Journal* **332**: 61–2.

Schwartz M, Savage W, George J, Emohare L. (1989) Women's knowledge and experience of cervical screening: a failure of health education and medical organization. *Community Medicine* **11**: 279–89.

Scotland, Scientific Services Advisory Group, Histopathology Subcommittee (Strong Report). (1988) *Report on Cervical Cytology Service in Scotland.* Edinburgh: Scottish Health Service Planning Council Scientific Services Advisory Group.

Scottish Health Service Planning Council, Scientific Services Advisory Group, Subcommittee on histopathology. (1977) *Working Group on Cervical Cytology Services in Scotland.* Edinburgh: Home and Health Department.

Scottish Office. (1993) *Report of the Inquiry into Cervical Cytopathology at Inverclyde Royal Hospital, Greenock.* Edinburgh: HMSO.

Scotto J, Bailar J C III. (1969) Rigoni-Stern and medical statistics: a nineteenth-century approach to cancer research. *Journal of the History of Medicine and Allied Sciences* **24**: 65–75.

Sharp L, Cochran C, Cotton S C, Gray N M, Gallagher M E (TOMBOLA group). (2006a) Enclosing a pen with a postal questionnaire can significantly increase the response rate. *Journal of Clinical Epidemiology* **59**: 747–54.

Sharp L, Cotton S C, Alexander L, Williams E, Gray N M, Reid J M (TOMBOLA group). (2006b) Reasons for participation and non-participation in a randomized controlled trial: postal questionnaire surveys of women eligible for TOMBOLA (Trial Of Management of Borderline and Other Low-Grade Abnormal smears). *Clinical Trials* **3**: 431–42.

Shaw W F. (1950) The birth of a college; the Lloyd Roberts Memorial lecture delivered at St Mary's Hospital, Manchester, on 10th October 1950. *Journal of Obstetrics and Gynaecology of the British Empire* **57**: 875–88.

Shaw W F. (1954a) *Twenty-five Years: The story of the Royal College of Obstetricians and Gynaecologists, 1929–54.* London: J & A Churchill Ltd.

Shaw W F. (1954b) The College, its past, present and future; the William Meredith Fletcher Shaw memorial lecture. *Journal of Obstetrics and Gynaecology of the British Empire* **61**: 557–66.

Sheehy A M, Coursin D B, Gabbay R A. (2009) Back to Wilson and Jungner: ten good reasons to screen for type 2 diabetes mellitus. *Mayo Clinic Proceedings* **84**: 38–42.

Sherris J, Friedman A, Wittet S, Davies P, Steben M, Saraiya M. (2006) Chapter 25: Education, training, and communication for HPV vaccines. *Vaccine* **24**: S3/210–18.

Shope R E. (1933) Infectious papillomatosis of rabbits. *Journal of Experimental Medicine* **58**: 607–24.

Shope R E. (1937) Immunization of rabbits to infectious papillomatosis. *Journal of Experimental Medicine* **65**: 219–31.

Shun-Zhang Yu, Miller A B, Sherman G J. (1982) Optimising the age, number of tests, and test interval for cervical screening in Canada. *Journal of Epidemiology and Community Health* **36**: 1–10.

Sigurdsson K, Sigvaldason H. (2007) Is it rational to start population-based cervical cancer screening at or soon after age 20? Analysis of time trends in preinvasive and invasive diseases. *European Journal of Cancer* **43**: 769–74.

Singer A. (1972) *The Effect of Physiological and Pathological Factors on the Cervix Uteri*. PhD thesis, Queen Elizabeth II research institute, department of obstetrics and gynaecology, University of Sydney, Australia.

Singer A. (1973) *A Study of the Cervix Uteri of Women in Prison*. DPhil thesis, Oriel College, Oxford University.

Singer A. (1975) The uterine cervix from adolescence to the menopause. *British Journal of Obstetrics and Gynaecology* **82**: 81–99.

Singer A. (1983) Sex and genital cancer in heterosexual women. *Journal of Reproductive Medicine* **28**: 109–15.

Singer A, McCance D. (1985) Commentary: the wart virus and genital neoplasia; a casual or causal association. *British Journal of Obstetrics and Gynaecology* **92**: 1083–5.

Singer A, Reid B L. (1976) Causes of cervical carcinoma: new ideas. *Comprehensive Therapy* **2**: 29–37.

Singer A, Stevenson M. (1972) Carcinoma of the cervix and herpesvirus. *British Medical Journal* **iii**: 290.

Singer A, Reid B L, Coppleson M. (1976) A hypothesis: the role of a high-risk male in the etiology of cervical carcinoma: a correlation of epidemiology and molecular biology. *American Journal of Obstetrics and Gynecology* **126**: 110–15.

Singer A, Shearman R P, Scott G C. (1969) Letter: contraceptives and cervical carcinoma. *British Medical Journal* **iv**: 108.

Singer A, Walker P G, McCance D J. (1984) Editorial: genital wart virus infections: nuisance or potentially lethal? *British Medical Journal* **288**: 735–7.

Slater D N, Rice S, Stewart R, Melling S E, Hewer E M, Smith J H. (2005) Proposed Sheffield quantitative criteria in cervical cytology to assist the diagnosis and grading of squamous intra-epithelial lesions, as some Bethesda system definitions require amendment. *Cytopathology* **16**: 168–78.

Southern E M. (1975) Detection of specific sequences among DNA fragments separated by gel electrophoresis. *Journal of Molecular Biology* **98**: 503–17.

Spratley J. (1990) *Disease Prevention and Health Promotion in Primary Health*. London: Health Education Council.

Spriggs A I. (1957) *The Cytology of Effusions.* London: William Heinemann Medical Books.

Spriggs A I. (1969) Automatic scanning for cervical smears. *Journal of Clinical Pathology* **3** (Suppl.): 1–7.

Spriggs A I. (1972) Population screening by the cervical smear. *Nature* **238**: 137–7.

Spriggs A I. (1977) History of cytodiagnosis. *Journal of Clinical Pathology* **30**: 1091–1102.

Spriggs A I, Boddington M M. (1970) *The Cytology of Effusions: Pleural, pericardial and peritoneal and of cerebrospinal fluid.* New York, NY: Grune and Stratton Inc.

Spriggs A I, Boddington M M. (1980) Progression and regression of cervical lesions. Review of smears from women followed without initial biopsy or treatment. *Journal of Clinical Pathology* **33**: 517–22.

Spriggs A I, Boddington M M. (1989) *Atlas of Serous Fluid Cytopathology: A guide to the cells of pleural, pericardial, peritoneal and hydrocele fluids.* Dordrecht; Lancaster: Kluwer Academic.

Spriggs A I, Bowey C E, Cowdell R H. (1971) Chromosomes of precancerous lesions of the cervix uteri. New data and a review. *Cancer* **27**: 1239–54.

Stening M. (1950) The extended radical vulvectomy of Stanley Way. *Medical Journal of Australia* **2**: 823–7.

Stern P L, Stanley M A. (eds) (1994) *Human Papillomaviruses and Cervical Cancer: Biology and immunology.* Oxford; New York, NY: Oxford University Press.

Stöppler M C, Straight S W, Tsao G, Schlegel R, McCance D J. (1996) The E5 gene of HPV-16 enhances keratinocyte immortalization by full-length DNA. *Virology* **223**: 251–4.

Stout N K, Goldhaber-Fiebert J D, Ortendahl J D, Goldie S J. (2008) Trade-offs in cervical cancer prevention: balancing benefits and risks. *Archives of Internal Medicine* **168**: 1881–9.

Sutton G C. (1997) Editorial: Will you still need me, will you still screen me, when I'm past 64? Breast screening policy is based on ageism. *British Medical Journal* **315**: 1032–3.

Syrjänen S, Puranen M. (2000) Human papillomavirus infections in children: the potential role of maternal transmission. *Critical Reviews in Oral Biology and Medicine* **11**: 259–74.

Syverton J T. (1952) The pathogenesis of the rabbit papilloma-to-carcinoma sequence. *Annals of the New York Academy of Sciences* **54**: 1126–40.

Thomas M, Pim D, Banks L. (1999) The role of the E6-p53 interaction in the molecular pathogenesis of HPV. *Oncogene* **18**: 7690–700.

Tidy J A, Mason W P, Farrell P J. (1989) A new and sensitive method of screening for human papillomavirus infection. *Obstetrics and Gynecology* **74**: 410–14.

Tierney R J, Ellis J R, Winter H, Kaur S, Wilson S, Woodman C B, Young L S. (1993) PCR for the detection of cervical HPV16 infection: the need for standardization. *International Journal of Cancer* **54**: 700–1.

Tighe J R. (1961) Brenner tumours of the ovary. A clinicopathological study. *Journal of Obstetrics and Gynaecology of the British Commonwealth* **68**: 292–6.

Threlfall A, Woodman C B J, Prior P. (1997) Breast Screening Programme: should the interval between tests depend on age? *Lancet* **349**: 472.

Traut H F, Papanicolaou G N. (1943) Cancer of the uterus: the vaginal smear in its diagnosis. *California and Western Medicine* **59**: 121–2.

UK Trial of Early Detection of Breast Cancer Group. (1981) Trial of early detection of breast cancer: description of method. *British Journal of Cancer* **44**: 618–27.

Unschuld P. (1985) *Medicine in China: A History of Ideas.* Berkeley, CA: University of California Press.

Wachtel E. (1964) *Exfoliative Cytology in Gynaecological Practice.* London: Butterworths.

Wachtel E, Plester J A. (1952) The vaginal smear as an aid to diagnosis of genital tract malignancy in women. *Journal of Obstetrics and Gynaecology of the British Empire* **59**: 323–6.

Wachtel E, Plester J A. (1954) Hormonal assessment by vaginal cytology. *Journal of Obstetrics and Gynaecology of the British Empire* **61**: 155–61.

Wakefield J, Yule R, Smith A, Adelstein A M. (1973) Relation of abnormal cytological smears and carcinoma of cervix uteri to husband's occupation. *British Medical Journal* **ii**: 142–3.

Walboomers J M, Jacobs M V, Manos M M, Bosch F X, Kummer J A, Shah K V, Snijders P J, Peto J, Meijer C J, Muñoz N. (1999) Human papillomavirus is a necessary cause of invasive cervical cancer worldwide. *Journal of Pathology* **189**: 12–19. Comment in: *Journal of Pathology* (1999) **189**: 1–3.

Walker P G, Singer A, Dyson J L, Oriel J D. (1983a) Natural history of cervical epithelial abnormalities in patients with vulval warts: a colposcopic study. *British Journal of Venereal Diseases* **59**: 327–9.

Walker P G, Singer A, Dyson J L, Shah K V, Wilters J, Coleman D V. (1983b) Colposcopy in the diagnosis of papillomavirus infection of the uterine cervix. *British Journal of Obstetrics and Gynaecology* **90**: 1082–6.

Walton R J, Blanchet M, Boyes D A, Carmichael J A, Marshall K G, Miller A B, Thompson D W. (Task Force appointed by the Conference of Deputy Ministers of Health, Canada). (1976) Cervical Cancer Screening Programs: the Walton report. *Canadian Medical Association Journal* **114**: 1003–33.

Walton R J, Allen H H, Anderson G H *et al.* (1982) Cervical Cancer Screening Programs: summary of the 1982 Canadian Task Force Report. *Canadian Medical Association Journal* **127**: 581–9.

Waugh N, Robertson A. (1996) Costs and benefits of cervical screening. II. Is it worthwhile reducing the screening interval from 5 to 3 years? *Cytopathology* **7**: 241–8.

Waugh N, Smith I, Robertson A, Reid G S, Halkerston R, Grant A. (1996a) Costs and benefits of cervical screening. I. The costs of the cervical screening programme. *Cytopathology* **7**: 231–40.

Waugh N, Smith I, Robertson A, Reid G S, Halkerston R, Grant A. (1996b) Costs and benefits of cervical screening. III. Cost/benefit analysis of a call of previously unscreened women. *Cytopathology* **7**: 249–55.

Way S. (1951) *Malignant Disease of the Female Genital Tract.* London: J & A Churchill Ltd.

Way S. (1954) Response to irradiation of carcinoma of the cervix at primary and secondary sites. *British Journal of Radiology* **27**: 651–5.

Way S. (1962) Exfoliative cytology, early carcinoma of the cervix, pregnancy and fertility. *Acta Cytologica* **6**: 547–50.

Way S. (1963) *The Diagnosis of Early Carcinoma of the Cervix.* London: Churchill.

Way S. (1967) Letter: cytological service and the Ministry. *British Medical Journal* **i**: 296–7.

Way S. (1969) Cervical cytology. *British Medical Journal* **ii**: 763.

Way S. (1980) Carcinoma metastatic in the cervix. *Gynecologic Oncology* **9**: 298–302.

Whynes D K (TOMBOLA Group). (2008) Correspondence between EQ-5D health state classifications and EQ VAS scores. *Health and Quality of Life Outcomes* **6**: 94.

Whynes D K, Woolley C, Philips Z (Trial of Management of Borderline and Other Low-grade Abnormal smears group). (2008) Management of low-grade cervical abnormalities detected at screening: which method do women prefer? *Cytopathology* **19**: 355–62.

Wilson J M G. (1961) Screening for cervical cancer. *Monthly Bulletin of the Ministry of Health and the Public Health Laboratory Service* **20**: 214–22.

Wilson J M G. (1967) Letter: cytological service and the Ministry. *British Medical Journal* **i**: 498–9.

Wilson J M G. (1971) The socio-medical problems of mass screening, in Riggott J M. (ed.) *The Early Diagnosis of Cancer of the Cervix*: A symposium held at the University of Hull on the 20 March 1970 as part of the 11th Annual General Meeting of the British Association for Cancer Research. Hull: University of Hull: 67–81.

Wilson J M G, Jungner G. (1968) *Principles and Practice of Screening for Disease,* public health papers no. 34. Geneva: WHO. Freely available at: http://whqlibdoc.who.int/php/WHO_PHP_34.pdf (visited 7 September 2009).

Wilson J M G, Chamberlain J, Cochrane A L. (1971) Letter: screening for cervical cancer. *Lancet* **297**: 297–8.

Wilson R M. (2000) Screening for breast and cervical cancer as a common cause for litigation. *British Medical Journal* **320**: 1352–3.

Wolfe C, Doherty I, Raju K S, Holtom R, Richardson P. (1992) First steps in the development of an information and counselling service for women with an abnormal smear result. *European Journal of Obstetrics, Gynaecology and Reproductive Biology* **45**: 201–6.

Wolfendale M R. (1991) Cervical samplers: most important variable is probably the operator's skill. *British Medical Journal* **302**: 1554–5.

Wolfendale M R, King S, Usherwood M M. (1983) Abnormal cervical smears: are we in for an epidemic? *British Medical Journal* **287**: 526–8.

Wolfendale M R, Howe-Guest R, Usherwood M M, Draper G J. (1987) Controlled trial of a new cervical spatula. *British Medical Journal* **294**: 33–5.

Woolley C, Philips Z, Whynes D K, Cotton S C, Gray N M, Sharp L, Little J, Waugh N R (TOMBOLA group). (2007) United Kingdom cervical cancer screening and the costs of time and travel. *International Journal of Technology Assessment in Health Care* **23**: 232–9.

World Health Organization (WHO). (2002) *Cervical Cancer Screening in Developing Countries: Report of a WHO consultation.* Geneva: WHO. Freely available at www.who.int/cancer/media/en/cancer_cervical_37321.pdf (visited 7 August 2009).

Wright T C Jr, Schiffman M, Solomon D, Cox J T, Garcia F, Goldie S, Hatch K, Noller K L, Roach N, Runowicz C, Saslow D. (2004) Interim guidance for the use of human papillomavirus DNA testing as an adjunct to cervical cytology for screening. *Obstetrics and Gynecology* **103**: 304–9.

Zhou J, Sun X Y, Stenzel D J, Frazer I H. (1991) Expression of vaccinia recombinant HPV 16 L1 and L2 ORF proteins in epithelial cells is sufficient for assembly of HPV virion-like particles. *Virology* **185**: 251–7.

Zhou J, Sun X Y, Louis K, Frazer I H. (1994) Interaction of human papillomavirus (HPV) type 16 capsid proteins with HPV DNA requires an intact L2 N-terminal sequence. *Journal of Virology* **68**: 619–25.

Zhou J, Sun X Y, Davies H, Crawford L, Park D, Frazer I H. (1992) Definition of linear antigenic regions of the HPV16 L1 capsid protein using synthetic virion-like particles. *Virology* **189**: 592–9.

Zhou J, Crawford L, McLean L, Sun X Y, Stanley M, Almond N, Smith G L. (1990) Increased antibody responses to human papillomavirus type 16 L1 protein expressed by recombinant vaccinia virus lacking serine protease inhibitor genes. *Journal of General Virology* **71**: 2185–90.

Zimet G D, Liddon N, Rosenthal S L, Lazcano-Ponce E, Allen B. (2006) Chapter 24: Psychosocial aspects of vaccine acceptability. *Vaccine* **24** (Suppl 3): S3201–9.

Biographical notes*

Professor Valerie Beral FRCP FMedSci FRS (b. 1946), epidemiologist, was born and educated in Australia with degrees in both medicine and surgery from the University of Sydney and a combined course in epidemiology and statistics at the London School of Hygiene and Tropical Medicine, where she was lecturer and reader. She has been the head of cancer epidemiology unit for Cancer Research UK since 1989. For further details on the million women study, the largest study of women's health, with one in four UK women who were aged 50-64 during the period of recruitment (1996–2001), see Beral (Million Women Study Collaborators (2003)). and http://info.cancerresearchuk.org/cancerandresearch/ourcurrentresearch/researchbygrantee/beral/ (visited 30 September 2009). See also Green *et al.* (1988).

Professor Saveria Campo PhD FRSE (b. 1947) studied at the University of Palermo, Italy, where she graduated *summa cum laude* in 1969. She obtained her PhD at the University of Edinburgh in 1973 and worked in the department of genetics (1973–76) and then in the department of zoology (1976–81). In 1980 she was awarded a Cancer Research career development fellowship and in 1982 she moved to Glasgow to the Beatson institute for cancer research where she led the papillomavirus research group. She obtained a Cancer Research life fellowship in 1984 and achieved professorial status in 1992. She moved to the institute of comparative medicine, University of Glasgow, in 1999, where she is professor of viral oncology. She was elected a fellow of the Royal Society of Edinburgh in 2006.

Professor Jocelyn Chamberlain FRCP FFPH (b. 1932) graduated in medicine in 1955 at St George's Hospital Medical School, University of London and pursued a career in epidemiology at Guy's Hospital (1961–68), the London School of Hygiene and Tropical Medicine (1968–73), and University College Hospital Medical School (1973–78), before moving to the Institute of Cancer Research, University of London, where she founded the cancer

* Contributors are asked to supply details; other entries are compiled from conventional biographical sources.

screening evaluation unit, funded by the Department of Health (DoH) research division, and directed it until her retirement in 1995, when she moved to Wales and became chairman of the South West Wales cancer institute until 2002. She served on numerous national and international committees, including the DoH standing subcommittee on cancer, the MRC molecular and cellular medicine board, the UKCCCR subcommittee on breast screening research (chairman), the board of the Faculty of Public Health, and the International Union against Cancer (UICC) core committee on cancer screening.

Professor Dulcie Coleman
MD FRCPath FIAC (b. 1932) qualified at St Bartholomew's Hospital Medical School, London, and trained in clinical cytopathology there under the supervision of Dr Gordon Canti and with Professor Erica Wachtel at Hammersmith Hospital(1962–64). She was appointed clinical assistant in in the department of pathology, Hillingdon Hospital, London, in 1964; became clinical assistant in the department of pathology, St Mary's Hospital, in 1965, appointed consultant cytopathologist there in 1972 and professor of cytopathology, Imperial College Faculty of Medicine (1988–98) until her retirement, later emeritus, and remains engaged in teaching and research.

Dr Lionel Crawford
PhD FRSE FRS (b. 1932) was senior scholar, then research fellow of Emmanuel College Cambridge (1952–58). After two years as a Rockefeller research fellow at the Virus Laboratory, Berkeley, and the California Institute of Technology, Pasadena, he returned to the Institute of Virology, University of Glasgow. He was subsequently head of the department of molecular virology at the Imperial Cancer Research Fund Laboratory, London, and then set up the ICRF tumour virus group in Cambridge (1988). His interest in papillomaviruses goes back to the early 1960s and continues to the present with forays into polyoma, SV40 and extensively into p53. He was awarded the Gabor medal of the Royal Society in 2005.

Professor Heather Cubie
PhD FRCPath (b. 1946) graduated in bacteriology in 1968, later receiving an MSc and PhD, all from University of Edinburgh. She has worked in either the University of Edinburgh (medical microbiology and dermatology) or NHS Lothian (Royal Hospital for Sick Children, City Hospital and

the Royal Infirmary of Edinburgh) since then, becoming a consultant clinical scientist in virology in 1993. Her specialist research interest is human papillomavirus (HPV). She is a member of the Scottish HPV national steering group and epidemiology and surveillance subgroup and also of the UK NCSP HPV special interest group. She became honorary professor of research and research management, University of Edinburgh, in 2006 and visiting professor of virology, University of Glasgow, in 2008.

Professor Jack Cuzick
PhD FMedSci (b. 1948) holds a PhD in mathematics and has been head of the Cancer Research UK centre for epidemiology, mathematics and statistics in London and John Snow Professor of Epidemiology at the Wolfson Institute of Preventive Medicine at Queen Mary, University of London since 2004. His current interests are in cancer epidemiology and clinical trials, with special interest in prevention and screening and he is currently involved in studies on the use of HPV assays for cervical screening. He discovered a method for sensing and processing biopotentials for early diagnosis of breast cancer (named on US patent no. 6,351,666 B1 assigned to the Biofield Corporation in 2003; for precursors, see Cuzick *et al.* (1998b)); received the Thomson's hottest research award of 2005/06 for scientists with most cited papers, the only UK-based author of 17 scientists selected worldwide; and has been president, International Society of Cancer Prevention since 2004.

Professor Nicholas Day
CBE FRSS FRCPath FMedSci FRS (b. 1939) statistician, later head of the unit of biostatistics and field studies, epidemiology section of the International Agency for Research on Cancer, in Lyons (1969–86), director of the MRC biostatistics unit, Cambridge (1986–89, honorary director 1989–99), professor of public health, University of Cambridge (1989–99) and MRC research professor of epidemiology there (1999–2004). He was chairman of the MRC committee on the epidemiology and surveillance of AIDs (1988–92). See Breslow and Day (eds) (1987).

Dr Ian Duncan
FRCOG FHEA (b. 1943) graduated in medicine at the University of St Andrews and trained in obstetrics and gynaecology in Dundee (1969–72, 1974–8), specializing in gynaecological oncology at Duke University, Durham, North Carolina (1972–74). He

was appointed senior lecturer, University of Dundee, in 1978, subsequently reader and honorary consultant gynaecologist/ oncologist until his retirement in 2007. He established one of the first colposcopy services in Scotland in 1974; has been executive member and subsequently president of the British Society for Colposcopy and Cervical Pathology (1985–88), the British Gynaecological Cancer Society (1988–91) and the International Federation for Cervical Pathology and Colposcopy (1993–96.) He has also served on the Strong advisory committee on the cervical cytology service in Scotland (1985/6), the intercollegiate working party on cervical cytology screening in the UK (1987), the NHS Cervical Screening Programme national coordinating network and its successor the NHS CSP, editing, drawing up and subsequent revision of guidelines for clinical practice and programme management (1989–97). He was chairman of the Scottish Cervical Screening Programme national advisory group (1998–2003).

Professor Ian Frazer
immunologist, jointly holds the patent with his late research partner, Dr Jian Zhou (1957–99), and was the commercial driver in the development of the vaccine for cervical cancer (*Gardasil*) by the University of Queensland team. He is head of the University of Queensland Diamantina institute for cancer, Princess Alexandra Hospital and was honoured as 2006 Australian of the Year, was inaugural winner of the Queensland smart state premier's fellowship (2006) and received the Balzan prize for international medicine. See interview by Robyn Williams in 2008 at www.science.org.au/scientists/if.htm; see also www.di.uq.edu.au/news-archive (both sites visited 23 April 2009).

Professor Lutz Gissmann
German Cancer Research Center, Heidelberg, Germany, was appointed to a postdoctoral position, later assistant professor, department of virology, University of Freiburg (1977–83); head of the German Cancer Research Center, genome modifications and carcinogenesis division, Heidelberg Germany (1983–); full professor (1986); chairman, applied tumor virology programme, German Cancer Research Center (1991–93); director of research, department of obstetrics and gynecology, programme leader for viral oncology and full professor, Loyola University Medical Center, Chicago, Illinois (1993–97); vice president of research and development, MediGene AG, Martinsried, Germany (1998/9);

honorary professor, King Saud University, Riyadh, Saudi Arabia (2008–).

Sir Muir Gray
Kt CBE MD FRCP FRCPSGlas FFPH (b. 1944) qualified at the University of Glasgow and trained in public health at Bristol. After house jobs he joined the city of Oxford as senior medical officer (1972–74); public health specialist, Oxfordshire HA (1974–91); director, health policy and public health, Oxford RHA (1991–94); Director of R&D, Anglia and Oxford RHA, then Anglia and Oxford Regional Office, NHS Executive, Department of Health (DoH) (1994–98); director of the Institute of Health Sciences, University of Oxford (1999–2002). He was co-ordinator of the national breast cancer screening programme, 1988–91; national cervical screening programme (1988–94); and Adviser, WHO (1984–91). He has been programmes director, UK national screening committee, since 1995, and director of clinical knowledge, process and safety, Department of Health, since 2004. See Gray (1997, 2004).

Dr Winifred Gray
FRCPath (b. 1937) qualified in Adelaide and trained in cytopathology with Dr Arthur Spriggs in the cytology department in Oxford. She took up a post in cytology at the Northampton and Kettering General Hospitals; was one of the first to have a full training in pathology at the Radcliffe Infirmary, Oxford, starting in 1969, under Dr Rosemary Ruse's married women's retraining scheme; was consultant histo/cytopathologist, Wycombe General Hospital (1974–88) and John Radcliffe Hospital, Oxford (1988–2002), where she set up a cytology training school for technical and medical staff, which closed on her retirement. She examined in cytopathology for the Royal College of Pathologists and served on their cytopathology subcommittee; was editor of *Cytopathology* (1998–2002) and on the BSCC council. The third edition of her textbook (Gray and McKee (2003)) is in preparation.

Professor Matti Hakama
statistician and professor of epidemiology at the University of Tampere, Finland.

Professor Harald zur Hausen
MD (b. 1936) studied medicine at the Universities of Bonn, Hamburg and Düsseldorf, working as a post-doctoral student at the Institute of Microbiology in Düsseldorf, assistant professor in the virus laboratories of the Children's Hospital in Philadelphia, Pennsylvania; senior

scientist at the Institute of Virology, University of Würzburg and as chairman and professor of virology at the University of Erlangen-Nürnberg, moving to a similar position at the University of Freiburg in 1977; and as scientific director of the Deutsches Krebsforschungszentrum (German Cancer Research Center) in Heidelberg (1983–2003). His special interest is in infection-induced malignancies and he showed the role of papillomaviruses in cervical cancer and discovered a larger number of novel virus types. He shared half the 2008 Nobel prize in Medicine or Physiology with Françoise Barré-Sinoussi and Luc Montagnier, recognized 'for his discovery of human papilloma viruses causing cervical cancer'. He has been editor-in-chief of the *International Journal of Cancer* since 2000. See also zur Hausen (2006).

Dr Amanda Herbert
MRCS LRCP FRCPath (b. 1943) qualified in medicine at St Mary's Hospital, London in 1968. Appointed as consultant cytopathologist and histopathologist at Southampton University Hospitals Trust (1982–98), she held a similar post at Guy's and St Thomas' NHS Foundation Trust (1998–2008), since when she works part-time in the same department. She is an honorary senior lecturer at Guy's, King's and St Thomas' School of Medicine. She chaired the Royal College of Pathologists cytopathology subcommittee and examination panel (1993–97) and was a member of council and/or officer of the BSCC almost continually (1984–2004). She has been editor of the Wiley-Blackwell journal *Cytopathology* since 2008.

Dr O A N (Nasseem) Husain
MD FRCPath FRCOG (b. 1924) qualified King's College Hospital Medical School and military service in the RAMC as a specialist in pathology, training at Westminster Hospital, London. He was the first NHS consultant in cytopathology in the UK in 1961 appointed to the Chelsea and Kensington Group pathological laboratories and in charge of the cytodiagnostic unit at St Stephen's Hospital, London, later Chelsea and Westminster Hospital (1961–91). He was co-founder and secretary, then chairman and ultimately president (1977–80) of the British Society of Clinical Cytology (BSCC). See Husain and Butler (1999).

Professor David Jenkins
MA MD FRCPath (b. 1946) studied at King's College, Cambridge, and then at the Welsh National School of Medicine, Cardiff. He was assistant lecturer in the department of pathology, Cambridge University, and then lecturer in pathology at Westminster

and St Thomas' Hospitals, London. He started clinical and laboratory research on the role of HPV in cervical and other cancers and precancer in 1984 with Albert Singer at the Whittington and Royal Northern Hospitals and continued at Nottingham as professor in pathology. He was a principal investigator on the MRC TOMBOLA trial of management of abnormal smears in cervical screening and became director of clinical research into prophylactic HPV vaccines at GlaxoSmithKline Biologicals based in Belgium from 2003 until his retirement in 2007. He remains an active scientific consultant to this vaccine programme and continuing evaluation and publication of the results of the large clinical trials he established on the HPV vaccine.

Professor Anne Johnson FRCP FFPH FRCGP FMedSci (b. 1954) trained in medicine in Cambridge and Newcastle and specialized in epidemiology and public health. She was in general practice (1978–83), registrar in community medicine, NE Thames Regional Health Authority (1983/4), lecturer, Middlesex Hospital Medical School (part of University Hospital Medical School since 1987, 1985–88); senior lecturer in epidemiology (1988–94), honorary consultant in public health medicine since 1998, reader in epidemiology 1994–96; professor of epidemiology (1996–), head of the department of primary care and population sciences, Royal Free and UCH Medical School (2002–), and director of the Division of Population Health, UCL (2007). She was visiting professor at the London School of Hygiene and Tropical Medicine (1999–2006). She co-directed the Medical Research Council-UK Centre for Co-ordinating Epidemiological Studies of HIV and AIDS from 1985 until 1999 and was principal investigator on the 1990 Wellcome Trust-funded first National Survey of Sexual Attitudes and Lifestyles (Natsal 1990) and on MRC Natsal 2000. She was a deputy chair of the MRC infection and immunity board (2004–07, a member of the Department of Trade and Industry expert advisory group, foresight detection and identification of infectious diseases project (2004–07), a member of the Department of Health specialist advisory committee on antimicrobial resistance (2001–07), a member of the working party on public health: Ethical Issues (Nuffield Council for Bioethics) in 2007. She is a member of the Board of International Society of Sexually Transmitted Diseases Research (ISSTDR) and a non-executive director of the Whittington NHS Trust.

Professor Leopold Koss
MD HonFRCPath (b. 1920) received his MD degree from the University of Bern, Switzerland in 1946. He was chief of the cytology service and attending pathologist of the Memorial Sloan-Kettering Cancer Center, New York (1952–70) and has been professor and chairman emeritus of the department of pathology, Montefiore Medical Center, Albert Einstein College of Medicine, Bronx, New York since 1973. His textbook, *Diagnostic Cytology and its Histopathologic Bases* (Koss (1961)) was awarded a *Citation Classic* in 1989. He was made honorary fellow of the Royal College of Pathologists in 1996. See also Koss (2007).

Professor Attila Lörincz
PhD (b. 1954) molecular biologist, inventor of the hybrid capture series of tests for HPV while senior vice-president and chief scientific officer at the Digene Corporation (later part of QIAGEN, Gaithersburg, Maryland). He has been professor of molecular epidemiology at the Wolfson Institute of Preventive Medicine, Queen Mary, University of London, since 2007.

Dr Elizabeth (Betty) Macgregor
OBE MD FRCPath FRCOG (1920–2005) qualified at Glasgow with house jobs at Glasgow Royal Infirmary and Western General Hospital. In 1958 she became a research assistant at Aberdeen in the department of obstetrics and gynaecology run by Sir Dugald Baird, who wanted a screening programme for cervical cancer established in the then stable population and she learned to take and interpret smears and to use the Papanicolaou staining technique; she was awarded an MD in 1963. The Aberdeen screening programme was one of the first in the UK and she established a punchcard system for calling and recalling patients. She visited GP surgeries to take smears, started to analyse them and study the epidemiology, publishing evidence after five years and encouraging others to follow. She was president of the BSCC (1980–83, Figure 1). See Anon. (2005); Richmond (2005); www.oxforddnb.com/view/article/96184 (visited 16 September 2009).

Dr Elizabeth Mackenzie
FRCPath DPH (b. 1934) trained at St Bartholomew's Hospital Medical School, London, and was consultant cytopathologist, Southmead Hospital, Bristol (1986–94; and head of the department of cytology, 1987–90, 1991–94); consultant cytopathologist to BUPA screening service, The Glen BUPA Hospital, Bristol (1994–2007). She was manager of the cervical cytology

screening programme for Bristol & Weston district, Frenchay district and Southmead district (later Bristol and district health authority (1976–94)); was chairman of the regional cytological committee (1984); established the South West regional cytology training centre for cytoscreeners, medical laboratory scientific officers (MLSOs) and pathologists (1990); was secretary (1983–86) and president of the BSCC (1994–97); chairman of the South West Association of Clinical Pathologists (1987).

Dr Joan Macnab
PhD FRCPath qualified and trained at the University of Glasgow. She worked as a research assistant in infectious diseases (1959/60), poliomyelitis (1960/1) and a memorable spell as research assistant to Professor Guido Pontecorvo (1962–67) where she later took up an MRC scientific appointment. In 1967 she joined Professor John Subak-Sharpe, Director of the MRC Institute of Virology, University of Glasgow. As senior scientist and research team leader she took early retirement in 1995. Her early love of genetics influenced her approach to virology research. She has been scientific adviser to Medical Research Scotland (formerly the Scottish Hospital Endowments Research Trust) since 1996.

Professor Glenn McCluggage
FRCPath (b. 1963) trained in medicine at Queen's University of Belfast (QUB) in 1987; has worked as a trainee and consultant in histopathology in the Royal Group of Hospitals Trust, Belfast, since 1988. He was appointed an honorary professor in pathology, QUB, in 2005; has published approximately 250 peer-reviewed articles and reviews in gynaecological pathology; and is president of the British Association of Gynaecological Pathologists (2007–10).

Dr Euphemia McGoogan
MPath qualified at Aberdeen University Medical School and trained at the University of Edinburgh department of pathology. She was a senior lecturer there and honorary consultant pathologist (1983–2004); and was pathology patient services director for the Lothian University Hospitals NHS Trust in Edinburgh, responsible for the largest combined morbid anatomy, histopathology and cytopathology service in the UK. She was medical director, Europe, for the Cytyc Corporation (2004–08) and has owned her own consultancy service since 2008. She chaired an inquiry into cervical cytopathology at the Inverclyde Royal Hospital, Greenock (1993). See www.

cancerscreening.nhs.uk/cervical/publications/nhscsp22.pdf (visited 27 January 2009).

Professor Anthony Miller MD FRCP FRCP(C) FACE (b. 1931) qualified in medicine in 1955 and specialized in internal medicine. He was a member of the scientific staff of the Medical Research Council's tuberculosis and chest diseases unit, Brompton Hospital, London (1962–71). He directed the epidemiology unit of the National Cancer Institute of Canada (1971–86), and was chairman of the department of preventive medicine and biostatistics, University of Toronto (1992–96). He was senior scientist, International Agency for Research on Cancer, Lyons, France (1997–99) and served as head of the division of clinical epidemiology, German Cancer Research Center, Heidelberg, Germany (1999–2003), and is currently associate director of research at the Dalla Lana School of Public Health, University of Toronto, Canada. He is principal investigator of the Canadian national breast screening study and he serves as a consultant to the early detection research programme, division of cancer prevention, National Cancer Institute, Bethesda, Maryland, and to the World Health Organization's programme in cancer control. He chairs the cancer risk management advisory committee of the Canadian partnership against cancer and is a member of its advisory committee on cancer control.

Professor George Papanicolaou MD PhD (1883–1962) qualified in medicine at the University of Athens, studied philosophy of biologic sciences in Germany with August Weisman, earned his PhD in zoology in Munich and worked in France as a physiologist. He was appointed as a technical assistant in the department of anatomy, Cornell Medical School, at New York (1913–61), and consultant to the Strang Laboratory. While preparing his 1933 monograph on the human female sexual cycle 'as revealed by vaginal smear', he noted abnormal cells from the cervix and later re-evaluated the vaginal smear for cancer detection at the suggestion of Joseph Hinsey in 1939. Dr Herbert Traut, from the department of obstetrics and gynecology at Cornell, collaborated with Papanicolaou on the diagnostic potential of the vaginal smear, later called the Pap test, published in 1943. Papanicolaou's *Atlas of Exfoliative Cytology*, appeared in 1954, with a revision in 1960. See Hinsey (1962); Michalas (2000); Sawin (2002); www.papsociety.org/index.html (visited 22 July 2009).

Professor Julian Peto
DSc FMedSci (b. 1945) graduated in mathematics from Oxford in 1967. He was a research scientist with Sir Richard Doll in Oxford (1974–83) and chairman of the section of epidemiology at the Institute of Cancer Research (ICR, 1983–2004). His Cancer Research UK chair is now held jointly between the ICR and the London School of Hygiene and Tropical Medicine.

Dr Catherine Pike
(b. 1920) graduated in medicine at the University of Glasgow in 1943; served in the Royal Air Force medical service (1944–47); and subsequently took medical house and registrar posts followed by marriage and life in Tanganyika (Tanzania from 1964) until 1960. She was a community physician (child health and family planning) at Guildford (1960–67) when she retrained in cytology at St Thomas' Hospital, London. She was appointed consultant cytopathologist, Royal Surrey County Hospital (1978–85); a member of the national coordinating network for the UK cervical screening programme; a council member, BSCC. Following retirement in 1985, she worked on a screening programme with Professor Jocelyn Chamberlain at the Institute of Cancer Research, Sutton until 1992.

Dame Rosemary Rue
DBE FRCP FFPHM FRCPsych FRCS (1928–2004), physician and regional medical officer (1973–84) and regional general manager (1984–88) of the Oxford Regional Health Authority, who set up a married women doctors' retraining scheme. See Rue (1967); note 35.

Professor Peter Sasieni
PhD (b. 1963) studied mathematics at Cambridge University before going to the department of biostatistics at the University of Washington, where he obtained a PhD. His post-doctoral post was with Dr Jack Cuzick at ICRF, Bart's, London, in 1989 and it was there that he started studying cervical screening and became involved in the National Coordinating Committee. He moved to Queen Mary, University of London as professor of cancer epidemiology and biostatiscs in the Wolfson Institute of Preventive Medicine in 2002.

Professor Albert Singer
PhD DPhil FRCOG (b. 1938) attended Sydney University, graduating in 1960, specializing in obstetrics and gynaecology obtaining membership of the Royal College in 1967. He had joined Dr Malcolm Coppleson, a clinical gynaecologist and expert colposcopists, and Dr Bevan Reid,

an outstanding cellular biologist, in 1966, obtaining a PhD from Sydney University (Singer (1972)). He moved to Oxford in 1970 on a scholarship to continue his work on high-risk women for the development of cervical cancer by studying women in a large London prison where evidence of clinical HPV as a aetiological factor became evident and was awarded an DPhil for this work (Singer (1973)); worked in Sheffield investigating possible genetic markers in women with cervical precancer while also building a large colposcopy unit (1973–81) and has been at the Whittington Hospital NHS Trust since 1981 as a gynaecologist as well as holding chairs in gynaecological research and molecular pathology at UCL. His unit in collaboration with basic science units at UCL has been active in both basic and clinical HPV research as well as examining the role of genetic markers for cervical neoplasia diagnosis.

Dr John Smith
FRCPath MIAC (b. 1953) qualified at the Middlesex Hospital Medical School, London, and trained in histopathology and cytology at St Bartholomew's Hospital, London, and in Bristol, where he developed a particular interest in cervical cytology. He has been consultant histopathologist and cytopathologist at the Royal Hallamshire Hospital, Sheffield, and honorary senior clinical lecturer in pathology in the University of Sheffield. He was appointed a consultant in Sheffield in 1987 and since 1997 has practiced exclusively in gynaecological histopathology and cytology there. He is director of the East Pennine cytology training centre, director of the Sheffield Cervical Cytology Service and lead histopathologist at the Sheffield Gynaecological Cancer Centre. He is currently president of the BSCC and past chairman of the panel of examiners in cytology of the Royal College of Pathologists. He is an associate of the General Medical Council and has served on advisory committees of the GMC, Royal College of Pathologists, BSCC and the NHS cervical screening programme. He is a consultant adviser to the governments of Singapore, New Zealand and Jersey.

Dr Arthur Spriggs
DM FRCP FRCPath (b. 1919) studied medicine at Oxford, Liverpool and Edinburgh and served in the Royal Army Medical Corps as a graded physician (1944–47). He joined the pathology department at the Radcliffe Infirmary, Oxford; in the haematology department under Gwyn Macfarlane he began

studying the cells of serous fluids, and his DM thesis (1952) became the basis of a monograph 'The Cytology of Effusions' (1957). He spent three months in the US and Canada studying the cytology of vaginal and cervical smears using the Papanicolaou method. On his return, with the assistance of Michael Boddington, he inaugurated the cytodiagnostic service in Oxford in 1958. He was consultant cytologist to the United Oxford Hospitals from 1960 until his retirement in 1984.

Professor Margaret Stanley
OBE FMedSci (b. 1939) attended the Universities of London, Bristol and Adelaide and has been professor of epithelial biology, department of pathology, University of Cambridge, since 2003. She has served on several research council committees and was a member of the Biology and Biotechnology Science Research Council (2000–03); a member of Spongiform Encephalopathies Advisory Committee (SEAC), which advises the UK government on prion diseases. Her research interests concern the biology of cervical epithelium and how and why cancer of the cervix develops; her current research focuses on mechanisms of host defence and the development of vaccines and immunotherapies against human papillomaviruses, the cause of cervix cancer. She has been on the editorial board of *Sexually Transmitted Infections and Reviews in Medical Virology* since 2007 and is a member of the council of the International Papillomavirus Society.

Mrs Marilyn Symonds
CSi FIBMS (b. 1947) commenced work as student medical laboratory technician in 1963 at Stoke Mandeville Hospital, Aylesbury, specializing in cytology. She became head biomedical scientist in cellular pathology at Stoke Mandeville Hospital (1989–2002) and honorary secretary of the BSCC (2001–04). She was appointed hospital programme coordinator for cervical screening, Buckinghamshire Hospitals NHS Trust (2000) and advanced biomedical scientist practitioner (2002).

Dr Anne Szarewski
PhD FFSRH (b. 1959) graduated in medicine in 1982 and has been a registered colposcopist since 1987. She joined the Imperial Cancer Research Fund (ICRF, Cancer Research UK from 2002) in 1992 and obtained her PhD in 1997 from the University of London. She has continued to work for the Imperial Cancer Research Fund and is currently clinical consultant, honorary senior lecturer in the

CRUK centre for epidemiology, mathematics and statistics at the Wolfson Institute of Preventive Medicine, Barts and the London School of Medicine and Dentistry, University of London. Since 2003 she has been the editor-in-chief of the *Journal of Family Planning and Reproductive Health Care* and has been on the board of directors of the European Cervical Cancer Association (ECCA).

Professor E M (Tilli) Tansey PhD PhD HonFRCP FMedSci (b. 1953) is convenor of the History of Twentieth Century Medicine Group and professor of the history of modern medical sciences at the Wellcome Trust Centre for the History of Medicine at UCL.

Professor Leslie G Walker PhD FBPsS FIBiol (b. 1949) holds the chair of cancer rehabilitation in the postgraduate medical institute, University of Hull, in association with Hull York Medical School. He has been chair of the research committee of Breast Cancer Care (2004–08) and serves on a number of committees, including the Medical Research Council college of experts since 2008 and the research committee of the National Cancer Survivorship Initiative (Department of Health). His membership of editorial boards includes the *European Journal of Psychiatry, Contemporary Hypnosis, Psycho-Oncology and Complementary Therapies in Clinical Practice*. He is a former co-chair of the nominating committee of the International Psychosocial Oncology Society (2000–03) and served two terms of office as chairman of the British Psychosocial Oncology Society (1995–99). He was a member of the council of the British Society of Experimental and Clinical Hypnosis (1991–96; 2002–05), the population and behavioural sciences committee of Cancer Research UK and the National Cancer Research Institute complementary therapies clinical studies development group (2004–08).

Mr Patrick George Walker MD FRCOG (b. 1949) has been a consultant gynaecologist, Royal Free Hospital, London since 1986. His University of London MD was on 'Human papilloma virus and its relationship with cervical intraepithelial neoplasia' (1985). He was president of the British Society for Colposcopy and Cervical Pathology (2003–06) and secretary general (2006–08) of the International Federation for Cervical Pathology and Colposcopy and has been president since 2008.

Dr Richard J Walton
(d. 1995) born and qualified in New Zealand. Having served with the Royal New Zealand Navy, he was awarded a British Empire Cancer Campaign Research Fellowship in 1949 and trained in radiotherapy at the Royal Marsden Hospital, Sutton, London, under Professor Sir David Smithers. After he obtained the DMRT in 1953, Dr Malcolm MacCharles recruited him to Winnipeg, and he was appointed as head of radiotherapy and medical director of the Manitoba Cancer Treatment and Relief Institute (1954–57); the first executive director of the expanded and re-named Manitoba Cancer Treatment and Research Foundation (1957–73); vice-president medical at the newly incorporated Health Sciences Centre, Winnipeg and a full professor in the department of radiology, University of Manitoba, Winnipeg (1973–79). He was chairman of the two task forces on cervical cancer screening programmes in Canada (1974–76; 1980–82). See note 48.

Professor Sir Stanley Way
FRCS FRCOG (d. 1988) qualified at the Middlesex Hospital, London; trained at Newcastle hospitals and with Papanicolaou in 1948–49, was lecturer (1968) in gynaecological oncology, University of Newcastle upon Tyne and consultant surgeon, gynaecological research department, Queen Elizabeth Hospital, Gateshead, a pioneering cancer unit and ran one of the five national cytology training schools. He delivered the Joseph Price Oration of the American Gynecological and Obstetrical Society on 10 September 1959 on 'Carcinoma of the vulva'; and was founder member, treasurer and then chairman of the BSCC. See JKR (1988); Husain (1988).

Dr J M G (Max) Wilson
Principal medical officer at the Ministry of Health and joint author with G Jungner, chief of clinical chemistry department, Sahlgren's Hospital, Gothenburg, Sweden, of *Principles and Practice of Screening for Disease* (1968).

Dr Margaret Wolfendale
MD (b. 1931) qualified at the Royal Free Hospital London in 1956; was appointed registrar in exfoliative cytology to the Oxford Regional Hospital Board in 1962. She worked with Arthur Spriggs and other colleagues to establish a cytopathology service throughout the region and participated in many research projects, particularly associated with cervical screening. She was consultant cytopathologist at Stoke Mandeville Hospital, Aylesbury (1981–96).

Professor Ciaran Woodman
is at the School of Cancer Sciences, College of Medical and Dental Sciences, University of Birmingham, Edgbaston.

Dr Jian Zhou
PhD (1957–99), patent holder with Ian Frazer (patent WO 1993/002184) for a method of providing papilloma virus-like particles which may be used for diagnostic purposes or for incorporation in a vaccine for use in relation to infections caused by papilloma virus, studied medicine at Wenzhou Medical College after the cultural revolution, taking a master's degree at Zhejiang Medical University where he became interested in pathology and in 1985, a PhD at Henan Medical University, where he became interested in molecular biology and virology for human papillomavirus (HPV) and cancer research, receiving his degree in 1994. He was a postdoctoral training fellow at Beijing Medical University; research fellow of ICRF tumour virus laboratory, department of pathology, University of Cambridge; NHMRC senior research officer, centre for immunology and cancer research, department of medicine, University of Queensland, Brisbane, Australia; assistant professor, head of papillomavirus structure protein laboratory, Loyola University Medical School, Chicago, Illinois; and Lions principal research fellow and head of the papillomavirus structure protein laboratory, centre for immunology and cancer research, department of medicine, Princess Alexandra Hospital, University of Queensland (1987–99). He received grants for some 20 research projects and 11 patents (1992–99). A memorial volume is freely available at www.scribd.com/doc/2740521/zhou-jianprefaces-Etc (visited 23 April 2009). See Figure 5.

Glossary*

ABC (1995, 2000)
'**A**chievable standards, **B**enchmarks for reporting, **C**riteria for evaluating cervical cytopathology', known as 'ABC', is the report of a working party set up by the Royal College of Pathologists, the British Society for Clinical Cytology and the NHS Cervical Screening Programme, chaired by Dr Amanda Herbert. First published in October 1995 in the journal *Cytopathology* and as NHS CSP publication no. 1, it had a second edition in 2000, edited by Jane Johnson and Julietta Patnick. Both editions clarified the existing guidance on reporting cervical smears along with proposed performance indicators and criteria for evaluating the performance of cervical cytopathology. The first edition specified a full review of all aspects of the screening history, including re-examination of previous cervical smears, but this was not included in the second edition, whose working party was chaired by Dr Jane Johnson (Wilson (2002)).

adenocarcinoma of the cervix
A less frequent form of cancer than squamous cell carcinoma, but is becoming relatively and absolutely more frequent. It is of glandular origin, usually arising from the endocervix and is more difficult to detect by cytology and colposcopy.

biopsy, loop
An electrified wire loop used to remove abnormal cells identified during colposcopy. The tissue removed is examined under a microscope to ensure that the abnormal cells have been removed.

biopsy, punch
A biopsy performed using a punch, an instrument to cut and remove a disk of tissue.

British Society for Clinical Cytology
Mary Egerton, Moira Murray, Freda Osmond-Clarke and Erica Wachtel, having attended the first International Congress on Cytology sponsored by the International Academy of Gynaecological Cytology in Vienna in September 1961 considered that Great Britain was lagging far behind the US and Europe in the development of the speciality and that a society would help to establish and promote the practice of cytology throughout the UK. Consequently, a meeting was held at the Royal Society of

* Terms in bold appear in the Glossary as separate entries

Medicine on 1 December 1961 to discuss the formation of a society. A working party chaired by C W Taylor (Birmingham) formulated statutes for a registered charity to promote the growth and development of clinical cytology in the UK and the organization of scientific meetings. Membership was open to all registered medical practitioners interested in cytology. See www.clinicalcytology.co.uk/membership/history.asp#background (visited 3 December 2009).

carcinoma *in situ* (CIS)
An epithelium which displays disturbed differentiation throughout its thickness, but has not invaded the basement membrane. Formerly classified as preinvasive cancer, later in the category of pre-malignant change along with severe dysplasia. See also CIN.

cervical intraepithelial neoplasia (CIN1, -2 and -3)
A cytology grading system describing the pre-malignant change of cervical epithelium characterized by a proliferation of undifferentiated basal cells extending varying distances from basement membrane to surface. **CIN1**: undifferentiated stem cells in lower third of epithelium (mild dysplasia); **CIN2**: undifferentiated cells in lower two-thirds of epithelium (moderate dysplasia); **CIN3**: a lesion composed of primitive basal cells in the entire thickness of epithelial cells (both severe dysplasia and carcinoma *in situ*). See Richart (1964).

cervical smear, smear test, Pap smear
A technique developed for use on women by Dr G N Papanicolaou in the 1920s, including a staining method named after him, to check the health of the cervix and detect early changes in the cells of the cervix, which may develop into cancer. A small disposable spatula (Figure 6) is used to take a sample of cells from the surface of the cervix, which are then spread onto a glass slide and sent to a laboratory to be examined under a microscope. The infected cells can be seen in Figure 4. This test was phased out in the UK by the end of 2008 and replaced by **liquid-based cytology (LBC)**.

condylomata acuminata
A papilloma consisting of central connective tissue cores of tree-like organization covered by epithelium displaying papillomavirus infection. The term condyloma refers to a clinically obvious filiform fungating papillomas of genital skin or mucous membranes and is infectious.

cotton-tail rabbit papillomavirus (CRPV)
Also called the Shope papillomavirus.

dyskaryosis
A cytological change in the nuclei of cells, which correspond to the abnormal cells seen histologically in **CIN**: mild (superficial), moderate (intermediate) and severe (parabasal and basal).

dysplasia
A reaction to damage to the epithelial surface of the cervix, which may disappear spontaneously or following treatment, as described by Reagan and Patten (1962). The term is more frequently used to describe precancerous changes now described as CIN and is still used in some places outside the UK. Mild, moderate and severe dysplasia correspond to mild, moderate and severe dyskaryosis and to CIN1, 2 and 3.

genital warts
A benign epithelial proliferation caused by human papillomavirus (HPV) almost always caused by types of the virus that do not cause cancer.

electrophoresis
A process by which molecules, such as proteins, DNA or RNA fragments, can be separated according to size and electrical charge by applying an electric current to them. Each kind of molecule travels through the medium at a different rate, depending on its electrical charge and molecular size.

herpes simplex virus (HSV-I and -II)
HSV-1 is responsible for oral infections ('cold sores') acquired mainly in childhood. HSV-2 is more often associated with infection in the genital tract and is transmitted by sexual contact. However, this separation is not absolute. HSV type-specific antibody tests can be used to identify past infection with a given antibody type using a monoclonal antibody blocking ELISA test (enzyme-linked immunosorbent assay).

human papillomaviruses (HPV)
A family of more than 200 viruses that cause various growths, including plantar warts and genital warts, both of which are filterable and easily transmitted. Genital warts are classed as a sexually transmitted infection (STI) acquired mainly through sexual contact, often called condylomata acuminata. These are soft and often occur in clusters, internally or externally. The virus may be present and transmittable in the absence of warts. Problems can result from untreated warts, which

can grow quite large, or, in rare cases, from infection of an infant during delivery. In addition, certain types of HPV are known to be 'oncogenic' and are associated with various forms of cancer, including cervical, vulval and anal carcinoma as well as certain types of head and neck cancer. See also **vaccine.**

hybrid capture assays
A technique used to detect and monitor viral infections. It involves hybridisation of a single strand of target DNA to specific RNA probes, with the hybrid captured on a solid surface and detected using chemiluminescence. It is more sensitive than conventional Pap smears for detecting HPV infection and the absence of HPV detection correlates with a lack of dysplasia. See also note 26.

hybridization
The amalgamation of two single complementary nucleic acid strands by heating to form a duplex, detected in a liquid or solid phase. Southern blotting and dot blotting are forms of hybridization.

Intercollegiate Working Party on Cervical Cytology Screening (1987)
Guidelines produced by a working party of eight under the chairmanship of Professor Frank Sharp, following the DHSS's approach to the RCOG to look at clinical aspects of cervical cytopathology screening programme in the UK. Representatives were from the Royal College of Obstetricians and Gynaecologists, Pathologists, General Practitioners and the Faculty of Community Medicine. Their recommendations included: effective cervical screening programmes in all district health authorities; every adult woman should be screened at three-year intervals (20–64 years) with no upper age limit for those never having a smear; all women should receive the results of their tests; and monitoring the outcome of actions and feedback be implemented (page 31).

interval cancer
Detected in the 3- or 5-year interval between test dates, where the previous episode was closed with no diagnosis of cancer.

koilocyte
A cell with a shell-like vacuole that looks 'empty' on cytological or histological preparations but contains mature infective HPV virus (high-risk or low-risk). See Ayre (1949); Koss (1987); Figure 4.

liquid-based cytology (LBC)
A technique to take cells from the cervix using a special brush, which is rinsed into a small container of preservative or the head of the

brush snapped off and put into the container. The container is sent to the laboratory, where the cells are put onto a glass slide. Liquid-based cytology fixes the cells immediately and removes blood and inflammatory cells. Introduced in the UK in 2000, it was recommended by the National Institute for Clinical Excellence in 2003 and replaced the **Pap smear** throughout the UK in 2008. The feasibility of **HPV** triage for borderline cytology, to correctly identify those women who need colposcopy, is supported by the introduction of LBC, which enables an HPV test to be carried out on the same cytology sample and to be restricted to those samples where the cytology result has proved abnormal. See also **cervical smear**.

Ministry of Health 1966 Circular

Mr Kenneth Robinson's press conference on 21 October was reported in the *BMJ* ((1966) **ii**: 1083) following the earlier Circular (Ministry of Health (1966)). The press release indicated the progress in the development of a cervical screening service (101 000 women aged 35 and over in England and Wales tested monthly in December 1966 compared with 39 000 in December 1964; 457 trained technicians in June 1966 compared with 150 in December 1964). Mr Stanley Way in a letter to the *BMJ* in February 1967 (Way (1967)) disputed the accuracy of these details and noted that the new pay agreement for GPs from April 1967 would include special payments for smear testing, although the funding of the expansion of the cervical screening services were to be borne by the ratepayers. Way described ministry involvement as likely to create 'a "ministry camel" (a camel being an animal that looks like a horse which was designed by a committee).'

NHS Cervical Screening Programme

Cervical screening programmes started in the NHS in 1964, although haphazard in coverage, and became a nationwide service in 1988 with a computerized call and recall system. The policy objective was to reduce mortality by regular screening (all women aged 20–64 every five years and those over 65 who have not had two consecutive negative smears in the preceding ten years (DHSS (1988): paras 2–4), although moves were made to 'rationalize' the service in 1982 by offering two screenings to women aged 22–35, as a result of the Committee on Gynaecological Cytology (Penfold (1982)). See note 155; see also Blanks *et al.* (2000); www.cancerhelp.org.uk/help/default.asp?page=9596#tests (visited 13 July 2009).

p53 (protein 53 or tumor protein 53)
A gene discovered in 1979 by Lionel Crawford, David Lane, Arnold Levine, and Lloyd Old, that responds to DNA damage by stopping the cell cycle and turning-on DNA repair mechanisms to fix the damage, which, once repaired, allows the cell to re-enter the cell cycle as normal. Sometimes known as the guardian angel gene.

Pap smear, *see* **cervical test**

papilloma
A benign epithelial tumour characterized by a branching structure.

papillomavirus
Small oncogenic DNA viruses that cause warty proliferations on epidermal and mucosal surfaces.

polymerase chain reaction (PCR)
A fast technique for making an unlimited number of copies of any piece of DNA and used to demonstrate the presence of HPV DNA. For the background to this 1986 discovery for which Professor Kary Mullis shared the 1993 Nobel Prize for Chemistry, see http://nobelprize.org/chemistry/laureates/1993/mullis-lecture.html (visited 4 June 2009).

Scottish cervical screening
Cervical screening was introduced in Scotland in 1960 on a limited scale under the NHS, although not introduced as a population-based programme. In 1978 committees were established by the UK Department of Health and a review was carried out in Scotland resulting in the Strong Report (Scotland, Scientific Services Advisory Group, Histopathology Subcommittee (1988)). A nationwide cervical screening programme was introduced in Scotland in 1988 and the NHS Boards and Trusts introduced computerized call/recall systems in 1988/9. Note: In July 1985, the Lothian Health Board put a freeze on smear tests because existing laboratory facilities were swamped with a backlog of 10 000 un-read slides. In response to public concern about the freeze, Edinburgh District Local Health Council organized a public meeting, jointly with the Edinburgh District Council Women's Committee, in October 1985, followed by the creation of an action group, the 'Cervical Smear Campaign' (see www.lhsa.lib.ed.ac.uk/catalog/pdfs/GD31.pdf (visited 3 February 2009)). In 1992 Dr Ian Duncan chaired a group to advise the National Coordinating Network on the management of 14 distinct problems, including the use of quality assurance and internal audit as well as managing patients with HPV and CIN. These

recommendations were reviewed in 1997. See Jordan *et al.* (eds) (1982); Mant *et al.* (1988); Schwartz *et al.* (1989).

Southern blotting method
A method for detecting the presence of DNA or RNA, using a radio-labelled probe, which permits the detection of a single copy of a human gene in a sample of DNA fragments, separated by size by gel electrophoresis, and named after Professor Sir Edwin Southern whose invention this was in 1975. The transfer from a gel to retentive paper (blotting with paper towels) facilitates the physical transfer of the nucleic acids.

vaccine (*Gardasil*, Merck/Sanofi Pasteur; *Cervarix*, GSK)
Following on from work done by Dr Jian Zhou on VLPs, Merck led the basic and clinical research programmes leading to the discovery and development of *Gardasil*, which was approved by the US FDA for clinical trials on women in 1997 and for use in humans in 2006 (and European Union marketing authorization). *Gardasil* protects against about 70 per cent of human papillomavirus-related cervical cancers (types 6, 11, 16, and 18, including two strains that are responsible for nine in 10 cases of genital warts). The *Cervarix* vaccine was developed by GSK using the baculovirus technology to produce VLPs for HPV16 and -18 with a proprietary adjuvant to give a strong immune response. This vaccine was introduced in the UK in a national programme in 2008 following the completion of successful clinical trials (phase 2 and 3) in 2006, with European Union marketing authorization in 2007. See note 3. Some disappointment has been expressed about the UK's choice of vaccine (Kmietowicz (2008)).

Wilson and Jungner's classic criteria for disease screening, report for the World Health Organization in 1968:

1. The condition sought should be an important health problem;
2. There should be an accepted treatment for patients with recognized disease;
3. Facilities for diagnosis and treatment should be available;
4. There should be a latent or early symptomatic stage;
5. There should be a suitable test or examination;
6. The test should be acceptable to the population;
7. The natural history of the condition, including development from latent to

declared disease, should be adequately understood;

8. There should be an agreed policy on whom to treat as patients;
9. The cost of case finding (including diagnosis and treatment of patients diagnosed) should be economically balanced in relation to possible expenditure on medical care as a whole;
10. Case finding should be a continuing process and not a 'once and for all' project.

See Wilson and Jungner (1968): 26–39; Sheehy *et al.* (2009); Andermann *et al.* (2008).

Index: Subject

Index: Names

Biographical notes appear in bold

Key to cover photographs

Front cover, top to bottom

Professor Albert Singer

Professor Margaret Stanley

Dr Lionel Crawford

Professor Jocelyn Chamberlain

Back cover, top to bottom

Professor Anthony Miller

Professor Jack Cuzick and Dr Amanda Herbert

Professor Heather Cubie

Professor Peter Sasieni, Dr Ian Duncan

Lightning Source UK Ltd.
Milton Keynes UK
UKOW042100250212

187890UK00001B/116/P

9 780854 841233